SHARRON DAVIES

AND JULIA THORLEY

Pregnant and Fit

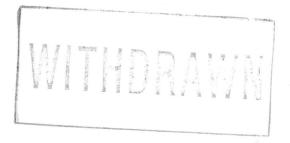

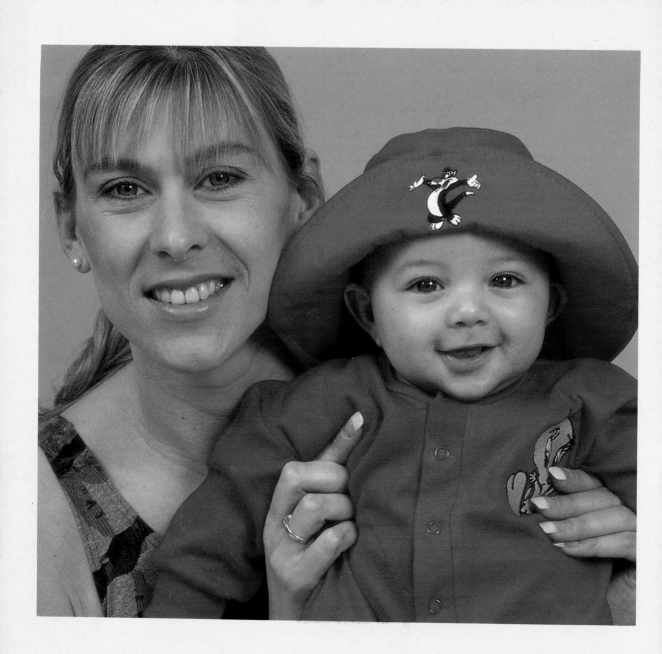

SHARRON DAVIES

AND JULIA THORLEY

Pregnant and Fit

Photographs by
Jennie Woodcock

PARTRIDGE PRESS

London   New York   Toronto   Sydney   Auckland

The Authors

Sharron Davies is Britain's most successful all-round female swimmer. She won a silver medal in Moscow in 1980 and has held over 200 British swimming records. She now works in the media, fashion and interior design businesses and is married to Olympic athlete Derek Redmond. Their baby boy Elliott was born in November 1993.

Julia Thorley is an author and editor of wide experience and has contributed to many publications, including *Baby* magazine amongst others. She is married with two young sons.

Acknowledgements

I should like to thank my family for their support both while I was pregnant and since, and for their patience while this book was being written; thanks also to all the staff at the Barratt Maternity Home, Northampton; to Lynne Hollingsworth, Senior Community Midwife/Supervisor, who delivered Elliott; and to Jennie Woodcock/Reflections who took the majority of the photographs for this book. *SD*

My thanks are due to the staff of Kettering General Hospital, and to all the many people and organisations to whom I turned for information. Thanks to my family, too, and in particular to Sam and Joe for their invaluable help in the research. *JT*

TRANSWORLD PUBLISHERS LTD
61–63 Uxbridge Road, London W5 5SA

TRANSWORLD PUBLISHERS (AUSTRALIA) PTY LTD
15–23 Helles Avenue, Moorebank, NSW 2170

TRANSWORLD PUBLISHERS (NZ) LTD
3 William Pickering Drive
Albany, Auckland

Published 1995 by Partridge Press
a division of Transworld Publishers Ltd
Copyright © Sharron Davies and Julia Thorley
Photographs copyright © Reflections Photolibrary
The right of Sharron Davies and Julia Thorley to be identified as authors of this work has been asserted in accordance with sections 77 and 78 of the Copyright Designs and Patents Act 1988.

A catalogue record for this book is available from the British Library.
ISBN 185225 2405.

Printed in Portugal by Printer Portuguesa

Pregnant and Fit was conceived and produced by Martin Marix Evans, Book Packaging and Marketing, Silverstone, Northamptonshire, England.

Design by Adrian Hodgkins Design, Oxford, England.

Typesetting by White Horse Graphics, Charlbury, Oxfordshire.

CONTENTS

CAUTION: Every individual is unique, and what is fine for one person may be unsuitable for another. Your personal requirements and the guidance of your medical adviser are more authoritative than anything suggested here, so do check with your GP before you decide to follow the experience described in this book. While every exercise has been designed with safety in mind, the publishers and authors cannot accept responsibility for any injury or damage suffered as a result of attempting them.

Chapter 1

WHAT THIS BOOK IS ABOUT

Being pregnant is one of the most important events of your life. This book is an account of my own experiences, and as such it offers some personal advice from someone who has been through it.

Obviously, the day you find out that you are expecting a baby is *not* the day you take up a new, strenuous exercise regime. But you will want to take care of the new life, and, by extension, yourself. As part of this you should be aware of how regular, moderate exercise and sensible eating can provide a good foundation for a healthy pregnancy – and life beyond that. If you make the effort to develop good habits for nine months, why go back to your old ways?

When I am not in serious training my exercise programme is planned but not too rigid, so if I have to go out for the day, I don't worry too much about missing a session in the pool. I exercise for about an hour each day. On three days of the week this will be aerobic exercise such as swimming or running, which works my cardio-vascular system, and on the other three I concentrate on muscle strength and tone, for instance by working out with weights. (When I was training for competitive swimming this increased to at least three hours a day, two of which were in the water.) In addition I also try to do some sit-ups and some stretching everyday.

When I was expecting Elliott there were some days when I did not feel like getting out of bed, let alone taking exercise, so I followed my instincts. If I felt awful, I eased up a bit, then took full advantage of my good days.

You might be thinking to yourself, 'It's OK for Sharron, she is a professional sportsperson. What about we ordinary people?' You are right, up to a point. I have been training since I was eight years old, so naturally I am used to listening to my body and responding to the messages that it gives me. But there is no mystery to it, no magic

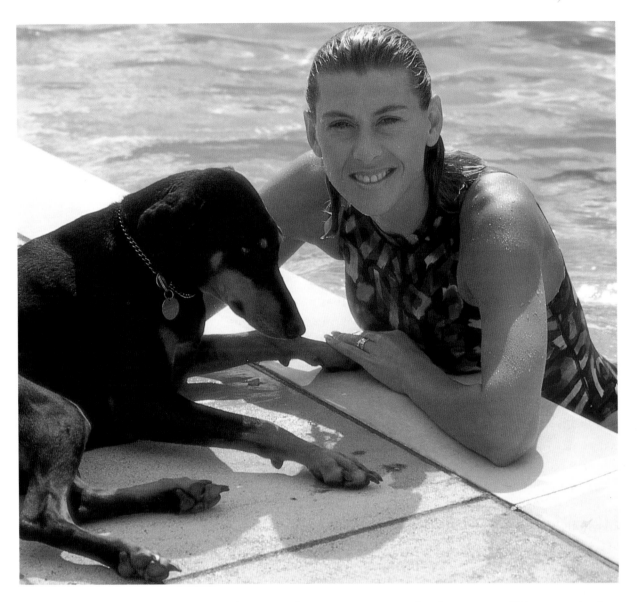

formula. Once you learn to trust your instincts you will be surprised how easy it is to decide what is right for *you*.

My main message is that pregnancy is not an illness and there is no need to retire from normal life just because of it. Certainly there are changes you have to make, but while you may stop running marathons you do not have to have to give up exercise altogether – indeed you *should* not. This book offers you one approach to having a pregnancy, one in which you stay fit, and which enables you to return to your pre-bump self as easily as possible.

Chapter 2

THE FIRST THREE MONTHS

Having a pregnancy confirmed affects different women in different ways. Some cannot wait to tell the world, while others prefer to keep it a secret for all sorts of reasons, perhaps to avoid a lot of questions or perhaps because they are superstitious. In many ways the first 13 weeks (technically speaking the first trimester) is the time when you are likely to be feeling your worst, but if no one knows you are pregnant you will not get any sympathy or understanding. You won't look pregnant yet, but you may find that you are tired and moody, nauseous if not actually sick, and generally out of sorts. This can be a very difficult time, but try not to worry too much. Listen to your body and just go with what it is trying to tell you. It may not seem like it on your darkest days, but it all passes and before long you will start to feel good again.

Moods

Your hormones will run riot as your body prepares itself for the months ahead, and you will probably find that your moods swing alarmingly from euphoria one minute to the depths of despair the next. Even if your pregnancy was planned, you might start to question your decision: I am not ready for this; I'm not cut out to be a mother; How will we afford it? What will it do to my relationship with my partner – not to mention my social life! Relax: this is normal. I found that one minute I was amazed and delighted at what was happening, then the next I was worried about it all.

What you *must* do is talk to your partner, because he is likely to be as confused as you are. Explain how you feel, so that he understands why you are bursting into tears for no apparent reason, and he will help you cope. If you find that you go off sex, your man will need reassuring that it is not him you have gone off. I found that I suddenly had great boobs, but was too tired to take advantage of them!

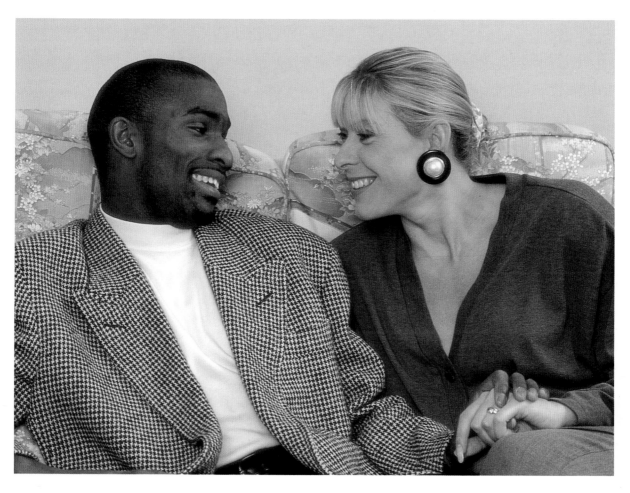

Making time to talk to each other about your problems, and his, is vital.

Morning sickness

There are two great myths about morning sickness: first, that it only happens in the morning, and second, that you are always actually sick. For me, there were some days when I found that I could not walk from the top floor of the house to the bottom without making a dive into the bathroom. I felt as though I was going to die – in fact on some days I wanted to, but I can now report that this feeling does not last, and that it goes as suddenly as it comes. Some people glide through their pregnancy without feeling ill at all, but most will feel nauseous at some time. Those awful waves that wash over you at the most inconvenient moments are all part of the hormonal changes you are undergoing. It's like having that morning after feeling without having had the pleasures of the night before.

Everyone who has ever had morning sickness will offer you a cure

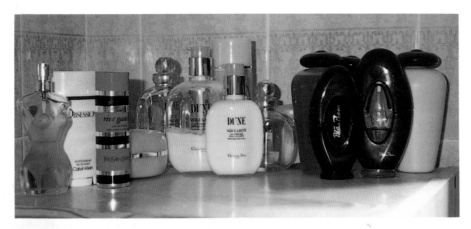

Morning sickness can strike at any time and can be caused by all sorts of things.

for it, whether it is dry crackers first thing in the morning, or a constant supply of chewing gum. Certainly it does seem to help if you can eat little and often, because, perversely, there is nothing worse than feeling sick on an empty stomach. Anything that refreshes your mouth is good too, such as peppermint tea or tonic water. Avoid fatty or sweet things as these are likely to make you feel worse. It might not just be tastes that upset you but also cooking smells or other aromas. For instance, I couldn't stand even the faintest whiff of aftershave for several weeks. But however awful you feel, *don't take any medicines unless prescribed by your doctor.* Even some 'natural' and herbal remedies are contraindicated too, so do check before you take anything.

Many pregnancy and child care books are full of helpful advice to rest whenever you can, or to try and start the day with a cup of tea and a biscuit in bed. Fine if you can, but if you already have children making demands on you or if you have to get to work on time this may not be all that easy.

The nature of my work means that many of my appointments are arranged up to three months in advance. On one memorable day early in my pregnancy I found I was booked to appear at the opening of a leisure centre, and obviously I could not back out at the eleventh hour. So I and my morning sickness got up at 5.30 in the morning to catch a plane from Heathrow to Glasgow, followed by a horrific taxi ride through the city. I was expecting only to have to make a short speech, cut a ribbon and then retire to a quiet corner where I could throw up in peace. But no. I was greeted by a sea of young faces expecting a much more active performance, including a spirited rendition of the okey-cokey. Needless to say, I survived – but I nearly didn't.

Then one morning after about three months, I woke up and discovered that I felt fine. This is the time when people say you start to 'bloom', and you might get the urge to buy maternity clothes and nursery equipment as the 'nesting instinct' kicks in (but don't feel disappointed if you don't!).

Exercising

If you are used to taking regular exercise you are not going to want to put away your training shoes just because you are pregnant, but if you are suffering from morning sickness or just feeling tired you will need to change your routine accordingly. This can be frustrating if you are determined not to let your pregnancy get in the way of your life, but try not to get too upset. Take it easy on your bad days, and capitalise on your good days. Even then, you might not feel like doing anything strenuous but a little gentle stretching will not do you any harm and may do wonders for your peace of mind. It is important not to slip into any bad habits at this early stage because if you do it will be all the more difficult to pick up where you left off once your baby is born. Try to keep up some form of exercise: at the very least go for a walk. Then as you start to feel better you can do a little more. Don't push yourself, but it is amazing how a little gentle exercise can lift your spirits. See Chapter 4 for some suggestions of exercises that you can do throughout your pregnancy.

Allied to exercise is the question of posture. The classic comic pregnancy pose is to stand with your hands in the small of your back, pushing your bump forward, and then to walk with an exaggerated waddle. I'm sure you don't need me to tell you how wrong this is! Stand like this and you will strain your back and overstretch your abdominal muscles. Instead it is important that you stand tall. Distribute your weight evenly between your feet, lift your ribs, tuck your bottom under and your bump in. When you sit down, don't slump but maintain this tall position, perhaps tucking a small cushion in the small of your back to help you. If you are working at a desk make sure that it is the right height for you, so that you don't have to stoop forward. When you have to pick up something from the floor, don't

Posture

bend and twist from your waist but instead bend your knees and if what you are picking up is heavy (and there is no one to do it for you), make sure you hold it close to your body to minimise strain. Of course, good posture is important throughout your life and not just when you are pregnant so establish some good habits and stick to them.

A word about miscarriage

Every mum-to-be worries about the possibility of a miscarriage, especially if she has already lost a baby. Most miscarriages occur within the first three months of pregnancy, which is one reason why many people keep the news to themselves for the first 12 weeks or so. If you have a history of miscarriage then you should be extra careful – talk to your midwife or doctor and get their opinion on what you should or should not be doing. If you are in any doubt it is better to err on the side of caution where exercise is concerned, but some people feel that if you are going to lose a baby then sadly you will lose it no matter what you do. It is Nature's way of saying that there was something wrong with the baby. Try not to become obsessive about it, but if you would like to talk to someone there are several organizations who will be able to help you and offer advice. See the reference section at the end of the book for some useful addresses.

Minor gripes and discomforts

As your pregnancy progresses you will notice all sorts of niggly little aches and pains, most of which will be quite normal but if you don't know what to expect you might be worried by them.

One of the most common problems experienced by pregnant women is backache. Try to alleviate this by adopting good posture when you are standing and sitting. Try not to slouch or to arch your back, and keep your weight evenly distributed. If you have to lift something off the floor, bend you knees and not your back. Try to rest with your feet up and your back supported. Some of the exercises in Chapter 4 will help you, but if the problem gets really severe talk to your midwife or GP for advice. You might also suffer from more headaches than usual. You can take paracetamol if you want to, but obviously it is better if you can manage without it. Do not exceed the recommended dose,

Correct posture is important during pregnancy. Don't waddle when you walk, and when you stand make sure that your weight is evenly distributed.

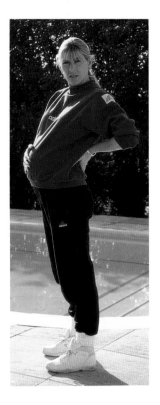

Don't stand like this . . .

and don't take anything stronger. Instead try some relaxation exercises and deep breathing, and do some gentle neck rolls. As with all these relatively minor 'side-effects' of pregnancy it is always worth mentioning them to your midwife, as they can be indications of something more serious, for instance raised blood pressure.

One of the early indications that you might be pregnant is that you suddenly need to go to the toilet much more than usual, and this is likely to carry on throughout your pregnancy. Towards the end when your bladder is really getting squashed you might find you have to get out of bed two or three times a night, but this is normal. However, if you experience any pain or burning sensation when you pass water, seek medical advice. Also if you think you might have thrush or other infection.

As your bump grows you might find that you become short of breath, but then by about week 36 (though sometimes not until later or even until labour has begun) your baby's head will engage in your pelvis. As it moves down into the bony part of the birth canal the pressure on your diaphragm is reduced, and you will suddenly find you are breathing easier. This is called 'lightening'.

The movements of your first baby will probably start to be felt by about 20 weeks, earlier for second and subsequent babies. When your baby first kicks you might not be sure that is what it is, because it feels like wind. Later, however, you will feel definite kicks and be in no doubt about it. Your baby might also get hiccups which you will feel as rhythmical 'jumps' inside your tummy. This is quite normal and nothing to worry about. Babies seem to develop a routine of sleeping and moving even before they are born, and some midwives like their patients to keep a 'kick chart' on which every movement is recorded. It is quite normal not to feel your baby moving for a while, and if you are busy you might not notice it anyway. But if you find that his movements become markedly less through a full day you should call your midwife or doctor.

From about 26 weeks you will occasionally experience Braxton Hicks contractions. These are tightenings of your abdomen and it will feel hard to the touch. This is caused by the early movements of the muscles of your womb, and the stronger your muscles the more you feel them. These are the forerunners of the contractions you will feel

. . . but stand like this.

in birth. Mums-to-be always want to know what a contraction will feel like, but it is very difficult to describe. The closest I can come to is to say it is like a very bad period pain accompanied by severe back ache. Painful contractions are often an indication that your labour has started, but it could also be signified by your waters breaking or a 'show', that is a slight loss of blood.

I suffered from cramp in my calf while I was expecting Elliott, particularly at night. If you get cramp you can try pulling your foot up with your hand or walking about. You might also get pins and needles in your hands during the second half of your pregnancy caused by compression of a nerve in your wrist. If this happens at night try raising your hand on your pillow. Again, it is normal.

It can be difficult to sleep when you are really big because you can't get comfortable, particularly if you are used to sleeping on your front. One of the things to look forward to after your baby is born is being able to lie flat on your tummy again!

Business matters

Even if you do not want anyone else to know that you are expecting, you must visit your doctor or midwife as soon as you think you might be pregnant. This is important so that you can ensure the best care for you and your baby. Precise details of antenatal care vary between health authorities, but you are likely to be given an ultrasound scan fairly early to determine your due date, and some blood tests need to be timed quite precisely to ensure an accurate result. More details of this can be found in Chapter 7.

In Britain, your doctor will give you a maternity certificate (MAT B1) which you will need to claim various benefits. While you are pregnant you are entitled to free prescriptions, and free dental care until your baby is one year old, so now is the time to get your mouth into good condition. There is an old wives' tale that says you lose a tooth for every baby you have, but there is no truth in this. However, you might find that you have bleeding gums and additional plaque forming on your teeth, so be scrupulous about your dental care.

If you are working, you should also notify your employer of your pregnancy as soon as possible, and check what your contract says about maternity leave. Obviously the precise details of benefits available will vary to a greater or lesser extent depending on where you are. Benefits are also likely to change, so do check carefully to make sure you claim everything to which you are entitled. When I was expecting Elliott the situation in England was as follows. (This information is for guidance only and should not be treated as a complete and authoritative statement of the law.)

Since October 1994 *every* woman who is working is entitled to 14 weeks' maternity leave. Leave must start no earlier than 11 weeks before your baby is due, but if you want to you can work right up until the week of the birth and take most of the 14 weeks after he is born. Women who have worked for the same employer for two years full-time or five years part-time, who are still working in the twelfth week before their baby is due, and provided their employer has over five employees, are entitled to 40 weeks leave. Again, this can start 11 weeks before your baby is due. If you wish to work longer you can, but you can't take more than 29 weeks off after your baby is born. In both cases you should write to your employer at least 21 days before you want your leave to begin, and enclose your MAT B1 maternity certificate. If you are taking 14 weeks' leave you do not need to give notice of your return to work unless it is earlier than the 14-week period, in which case you must give your employer seven days' written notice. If you are entitled to 40 weeks' leave, your employer will write to you while you are off work and ask when you intend to return. You must reply in writing within 14 days or you will lose your right to return. You should write to your employer at least 21 days before your planned return to confirm the exact date.

Your local Social Security office will be able to provide you with full details of what provisions the state makes for expectant mothers, and the sooner you put in any claims the better it is because any delay might mean you lose out. The following brief outline gives you some idea of what benefits are currently available.

Statutory Maternity Pay (SMP): a weekly payment made to you by your employer, based on the length of your employment and your earnings. You do not have to be intending to return to work to get it. You can claim SMP if you have been in the same job without a break for at least 26 weeks including and ending with the 15th week before the week your baby is due (called the qualifying week) *and* if your

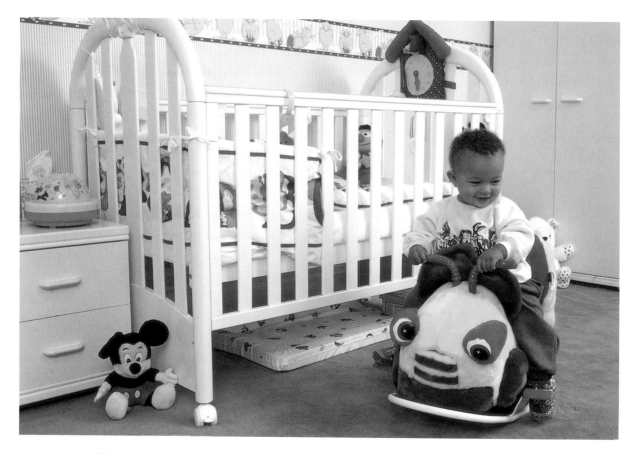

average weekly earnings were at or above the lower earnings limit
(at which you have to start paying National Insurance contributions).
You might also be entitled to it if your pregnancy caused you to be
dismissed before the qualifying week, or if your baby was born earlier
than this. SMP can be paid for up to 18 weeks.

Maternity Allowance: can be claimed by those women who are not
entitled to SMP either because they are self-employed or because they
have recently changed jobs. To claim this you must have paid enough
Class 1 or Class 2 NI contributions in a specified qualifying period. It
can be paid for 18 weeks. You get paid a flat rate, with extra if you
support another adult. It wasn't until we were researching this book
that I realised that as a self-employed person I could have claimed
this benefit. It provides quite a substantial sum which whilst not
replacing your normal income completely is nevertheless a very useful
regular contribution.

Sickness benefit: might be payable if you cannot get SMP or Maternity

*Equipping a nursery
is a costly business.*

Which benefit?

It is important that you claim everything to which you are entitled, as soon as you can. To find out what the current situation is, contact your local Social Security office (listed in the phone book under 'Social Security' or 'Benefits Agency', or for National Insurance matters 'Contributions Agency'). Some leaflets are also available in post offices or Employment Service Jobcentres. If you cannot find any of these leaflets locally, write to the Health Publications Unit, No 2 Site, Heywood Stores, Manchester Road, Heywood, Lancashire OL10 2PZ. All these leaflets are free.

AB11:   *Help with NHS costs*

CH1:   *Child benefit*

D11:   *NHS dental treatment*

FB2:   *Which benefit?*

FB27:   *Bringing up children?*

FB8:   *Babies and benefits*

NI16:   *Sickness benefit*

NI17A: *A guide to maternity benefits*

P11:   *NHS prescriptions*

SB16:   *Guide to the Social Fund*

Allowance, for the period beginning six weeks before the week the baby is expected until two weeks after the date of birth.

The Social Fund: helps people with expenses which are difficult to pay for out of regular income and does not depend on NI contributions.

Maternity Payment: one-off, non-repayable sum to help towards the expense of a new baby might be available if you or your partner is getting Income Support, Family Credit or Disability Working Allowance.

Free milk and vitamins: if you are claiming Income Support, you and children under five can claim for this. If you are receiving Family Credit and have a child under one who is not being breastfed, you can buy reduced priced dried baby milk from your maternity or child health clinic.

Child Benefit: a tax-free weekly cash payment that can be claimed by nearly everyone caring for children, regardless of income or NI contributions. It is payable for each child under 16 (and children aged 16, 17 or 18 if they are still in full-time education up to and including GCE A-level standard or equivalents).

Chapter 3

DIET AND NUTRITION

The best kind of diet for anyone, whatever stage of life they are at, is a balanced diet, which means taking a good selection of food from across the four food groups. When you are pregnant you have to take even more care with your diet than you might otherwise do, because everything you eat will also affect your unborn baby. However, this doesn't mean that you have to become an overnight expert on food additives and vitamins. Just use your common sense and have as varied a diet as you can.

What to eat . . .

There are four main food groups. The first group contains the starchy foods, and includes bread, rice, pasta, cereals and some vegetables such as potatoes and yams. These provide fibre, protein, energy and some vitamins and minerals, and are the foods that will fill you up. The second group is dairy foods, that is milk, cheese, yogurt, and these foods are essential for putting calcium, protein, vitamins and minerals into your diet. The third group contains those foods which provide protein, that is meat, fish, eggs, nuts and beans. Finally, fruit and vegetables provide vitamins A and C, folic acid, potassium, iron and fibre.

Try to include something from each group with every meal. For instance, start your day with a bowl of 'fruit and fibre'-type cereals topped with milk and followed by a slice of wholemeal toast. For lunch you might choose a tuna fish sandwich made with wholemeal bread, an apple and a glass of milk. Then for your evening meal, meat or fish with vegetables and a starch filler would be ideal.

It is important to try to have some breakfast to get you off to a good start for the day. A bowl of cereals is a particularly good idea because not only do you have the calcium in the milk but you also have the fibre in the cereals. Constipation (or, in extreme cases, piles) can be a

Healthy eating is essential in pregnancy – and throughout your life.

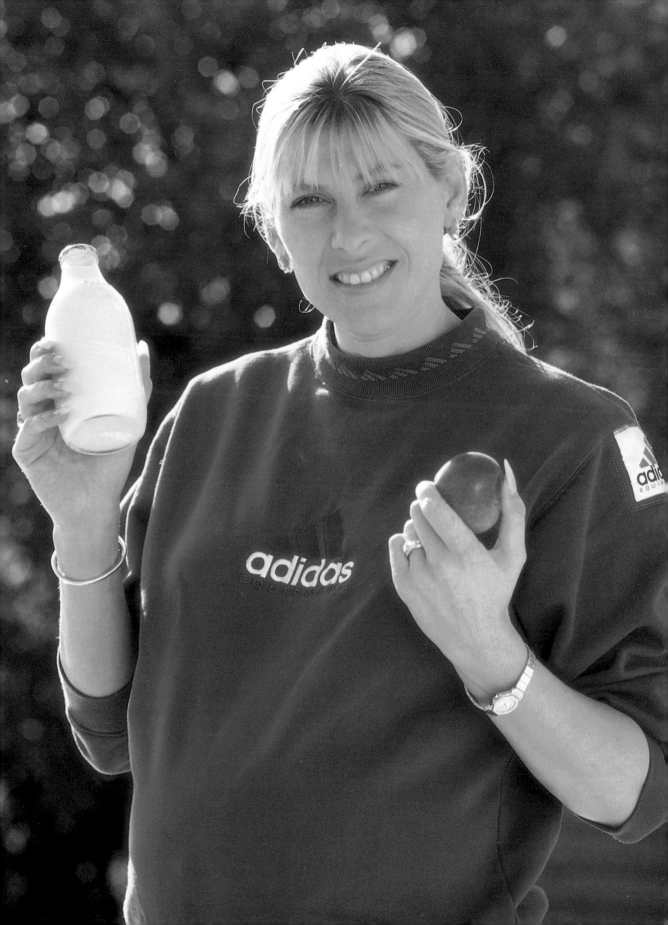

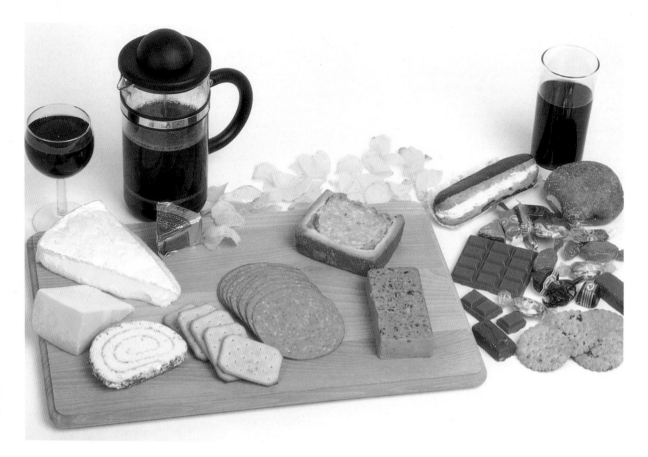

problem during pregnancy, but a diet that includes plenty of fibre will help to keep this at bay. If you find your digestive system does get a bit sluggish, increase the amount of wholemeal cereal and fruit and veg in your diet rather than reaching for a proprietary laxative. As with all medication, you *must* talk to your doctor before taking anything.

Your haemoglobin level will be checked regularly as part of your routine blood tests, and you may be advised to take a prescribed iron supplement, often combined with folic acid. Folic acid is one of the B vitamins, and has been the focus of much attention recently. A large-scale study indicated that it can be useful in preventing spina bifida, and the Department of Health now recommends that mothers who have already conceived a baby with spina bifida should take a folic acid supplement before they become pregnant again and possibly during the first 12 weeks.

As you will be taking advantage of free dental treatment, your

Foods to avoid during your pregnancy . . .

20

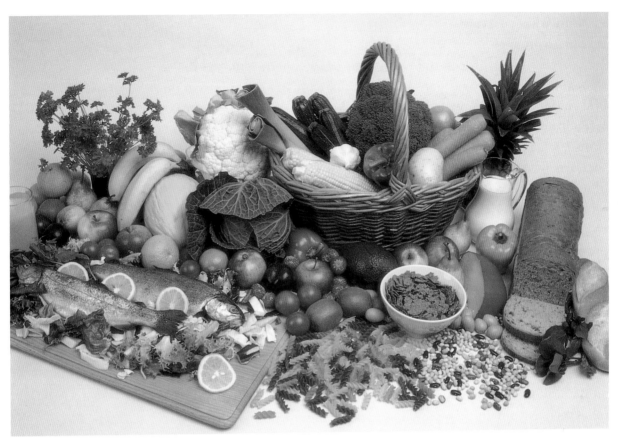

. . . and a selection of foods that are always good for you.

dentist should pick up any calcium deficiency. Incidentally, if you do need any dental treatment make sure you remind your dentist that you are pregnant if it is not obvious, because he or she may not know if he has a receptionist or dental nurse who handles all the paperwork. You should not have any x-rays and some anaesthetics are best avoided.

If you enjoy a balanced and varied diet you should not need to take any nutritional supplements unless advised to do so by your doctor. If you are a vegetarian you might be missing out on iron-rich foods, so boost your vitamin C intake to increase your absorption by eating more citrus fruits and leafy vegetables. If you are a strict vegan and therefore excluding dairy products you will need to take a supplement to boost the level of calcium in your diet. Also, vitamin B12 is only available in animal foods, so you may need to take a supplement of this too. Your doctor will advise you if this is likely to be the case.

. . . and what to avoid

It seems as though there is always some food scare or other in the news, so it can be difficult to be sure that what you are eating is the right thing. There are fashions in this as there are in everything, so the best thing to do is simply to be aware of the latest recommendations but not to let your diet occupy your every waking moment. For instance, when Julia was pregnant with her first baby, one of the foods that was recommended as good for pregnant women was liver because of its high iron content, but by the time her second baby was due this had been moved to the list of things to avoid because its high level of vitamin A is thought to have a toxic effect on the unborn baby. Imported soft cheeses which might be made from unpasteurised milk, all types of pâté, under-cooked meat and eggs, and ready-prepared salads are also currently on the list of foods to be avoided. The only advice that doesn't change is to use your common sense, and not to eat anything to excess.

As well as the four food groups outlined above, there are also, of course, sugary foods. Go easy on the sugar because too much can pile on the weight and can cause tooth decay. Cut down on fatty foods, too. Obviously no one is saying that you shouldn't eat anything unhealthy during your pregnancy because that is unrealistic, and the occasional bar of chocolate is not going to do you any harm. I did not exclude fat and sugar from my diet totally. Just be sensible.

There is a condition known as gestational diabetes in which a woman can develop diabetes as a result of being pregnant, and which may or may not go away once the baby is born. One of the things that is tested for in your urine sample at your routine antenatal check-ups is your sugar level, so if you do develop diabetes your GP will detect it before you notice any symptoms yourself.

While you are pregnant and making a conscious effort to eat a healthy diet you will develop some very good habits, not only in what you choose to eat, but also in what you leave out. This is an ideal opportunity to make these beneficial changes *for good*. If you can make the effort for nine months, why go back to your old ways once your baby is born? Healthy eating can become an automatic way of life. Similarly, if you have given up smoking during your pregnancy and cut back on your drinking, then keep it up. It is obviously better

Table 1 – How your pregnancy weight gain is made up.

	pounds
Baby's weight	7–7½
Placenta	1¼–1½
Amniotic fluid	2
Uterus	2
Breasts	1½–2
Extra blood volume	4
Stored fat and protein	4–7
Increased tissue fluid	4
Approximate total gain	30

Table 2 – How your baby grows.

12 weeks	1 oz
18 weeks	7 oz
24 weeks	1 lb
28 weeks	2 lb
32 weeks	3 lb 4 oz
36 weeks	5 lb 4 oz
40 weeks	7 lb

if you can give up alcohol altogether while you are pregnant, but the occasional glass of wine probably won't do either you or your baby any harm. *But definitely no smoking.* It has been shown that there is a link between smoking in pregnancy and cot death. Studies would seen to indicate that by eliminating smoking, putting a baby to sleep on his back, and ensuring that he is not kept too warm, the risk of cot death is cut dramatically.

Weight gain

If you are used to being a svelte size 10 it comes as an awful shock when you start to lose sight of your feet! Years ago people used to say that expectant women were 'eating for two', and while this is true up to a point it does not mean that you can get away with eating twice as much as you normally do.

When you first visit your GP or midwife for antenatal care you will be weighed. After that practice seems to vary from surgery to surgery, but you will probably be asked to hop on the scales every now and then just to make sure that all is well. This is yet another aspect of being pregnant about which it is easy to be over-anxious, particularly if you were very conscious of what you weighed in your pre-bump days. If you are used to trying not to put on any extra pounds it can be depressing watching the scales go up, but tell yourself that it is the baby, not you, and don't dwell on it.

You will need extra energy – and therefore extra calories – to meet your baby's needs and to store fat in preparation for breastfeeding, but your body will not need as much extra as you might think because your basal metabolic rate, that is the speed at which your body uses energy, will go down, especially towards the end of your pregnancy. On average a pregnant women only needs an extra 200 calories per day in the final three months, but *don't* get out your calorie charts. Be sensible and have an extra sandwich or a piece of fruit if you get hungry rather than another slice of chocolate cake. Try smaller meals more often to keep up your energy levels, and concentrate on foods that are high in nutrients but low in sugar and fat. Towards the end of your pregnancy when your stomach is being squashed upwards you might suffer from heartburn so smaller meals will be more comfortable. Even so, don't be tempted to snack on biscuits. Keep making the

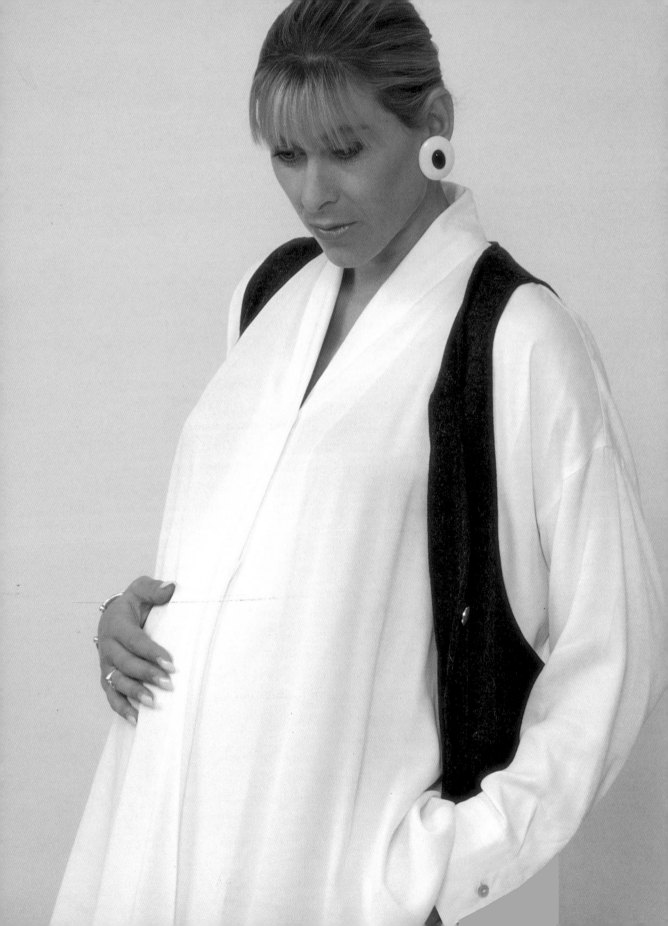

healthy choices. You might also begin to feel nauseous again depending on how your baby is lying, because there is so little room for your stomach.

The average weight gain during pregnancy is about 25–30 lb (11.25–13.5 kg), but this is *only* an average and you should not be perturbed if you put on more or less than this. Your midwife will notice if your weight gain is not as expected and will advise you if she thinks you need to change your diet in any way. You might not put on any weight in the first three months if you have been suffering from morning sickness and have been off your food, but once you are over that you will probably put on about 2 lb a week, slowing to 1 lb a week towards the end of your pregnancy. If this sounds like an awful lot, don't forget that an average newborn baby weighs about 7 lb. You can expect to lose about two-thirds of this extra weight within two weeks of delivery, and provided you are sensible about your diet and fitness, you will soon return to your pre-pregnancy weight. *Yes you will!* Don't allow the fact that you have had a baby to become an excuse for getting fat and flabby.

Cravings

A yearning for peculiar foods is a well-known 'side-effect' of being pregnant, although not everyone is affected. Some people believe that these cravings are your body's way of telling you that your diet is missing something. However, don't sit in front of the TV with 2 lb of jelly-beans and tell yourself *that* is a craving. If you find you have the urge to eat a non-food item such as coal (a condition known as pica), you should talk to your doctor. But as long as you don't overdo it, there is no harm in indulging your craving for pickled walnuts, beetroot and banana sandwiches, or whatever. It might be amusing to the rest of the household, but it is unlikely to do you any harm.

You can expect to put on about two stones by the end of your pregnancy.

Chapter 4

PHYSICAL EXERCISE AND WELL-BEING

I have already said that keeping physically fit is good for your body and your mind, but when you are pregnant you also have an extra incentive to take some exercise. If you are in good shape you will be able to cope better with the exertion and pain encountered during labour, and you will recover more quickly, too. Exercises done during pregnancy are done not to build muscle tone but rather as part of an overall health regime that will keep your body fit and your mind alert.

Obviously pregnancy is not the time to take up a new sport or to launch yourself into some energetic schedule, but if you are already used to taking part in some form of sport there is no need to give it up. As your pregnancy progresses your common sense will tell you when you need to ease up a little. Just listen to your body. High impact sports such as aerobics classes or long-distance running are best avoided, but there is no reason why you cannot carry on doing your normal fitness routine as long as you are sensible and don't push yourself too far. Don't expect to maintain the same levels as you achieved in your pre-pregnancy days, but do what you can and as much as you can for as long as you feel happy. Only you can say what is right for you.

Exercises

The following exercises are a selection of those that I did when I was expecting Elliott. Some are variations on a theme of stretching and others are more straightforward exercises.

The best position for any exercise that you do standing up is to position your feet apart, bend your knees slightly, tuck your tail in and keep your back straight. This ensures that your weight is evenly distributed and lessens the strain on your back and joints. There are also some exercises which you can do with your partner, and details of

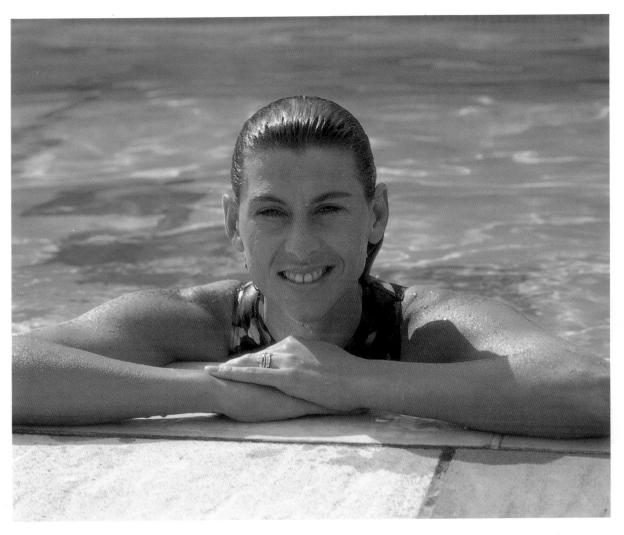

these are given in Chapter 9, while in Chapter 8 you can see the suggestions I make for post-natal exercises.

Exercising three times a week is very beneficial. Perhaps you could use a swimming pool one day and then on the next you could do the land-based exercises outlined below or do your normal sport. You should be able to work through all the exercises here fairly quickly, but if this proves to be too much for you try to do a different selection of exercises each time so that you do them all in rotation. When I was pregnant I swam three or four times a week for between 40 minutes and an hour, which for me meant I covered 2,500-3,000 metres. Obviously you wouldn't be expected to do this much, but 30 lengths or whatever you feel happy with is fine.

EXERCISE BIKE

An exercise bike is an excellent piece of equipment because it allows you to have quite a strenuous work-out without putting any strain on your joints. You can use one at a gym, or if you are lucky enough to have one at home park it in front of the telly and you won't even realise you are exercising.

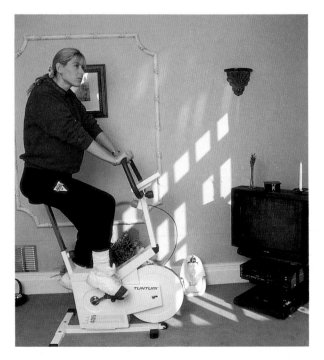

Although it is a static piece of equipment it provides an excellent work-out for the muscles of your bottom and legs, without the risks that go with cycling on the road. You do not have to do battle with other road users, there are no bumps and pot-holes, you are not going to fall off and you're not breathing in lungfuls of polluted air. It is also a low-impact exercise. I found my exercise bike very useful and continued to use it right to the end of my pregnancy. A 20-30 minute work-out is enough for a normal routine, and if you can cope quite comfortably with this during your pregnancy then rather than reduce the time you are exercising lower the resistance so that you are still doing the same amount of exercise but the workload is reduced. Don't over do it, however, and if you do get tired easily then obviously you should reduce the length of time you spend on the bike.

You are in control on a bike and can choose whatever level is comfortable. You can hold on to the handle bars or not, whatever you feel happiest with. Some bikes come with a rowing action and while these are good machines in their own way, they are perhaps not quite so good when you are pregnant. They are not very comfortable when you have a large bump in the way and you might not find it so easy to control what you are doing.

As well as working on your muscles cycling is also excellent cardiovascular exercise, getting oxygen into your blood. This is good for you and good for your baby who is, after all, depending on the same circulation.

It should not be difficult to find 20-30 minutes a day to use a bike, particularly towards the end of your pregnancy when you have given up work and are at home all day, and this is an example of a habit you can get into during your pregnancy and keep up afterwards. It all helps you to regain your pre-bump level of fitness.

One tip: the seat of an exercise bike is not designed for comfort at the best of times so you might want to add some padding as you get bigger because of all the extra weight pressing on your coccyx.

WORKING WITH WEIGHTS

1. DUMB-BELL CURLS

I am using dumb-bells here, but if you don't have any you can still do this exercise by substituting two cans of beans or any other two objects you have to hand that are equally weighted and easy to hold. This exercise tones up the front of your arms (biceps) and the back (triceps) which is the bit that wobbles!

Standing comfortably, slowly raise and lower the dumb-bell in alternate hands. Keep your elbows still or you will use your shoulder muscles, too. This should be a slow, controlled squeeze, so resist the temptation to swing the dumb-bells upwards. Try to visualise what is happening to your muscles. If you keep your hands facing forwards all the time you will exercise your biceps; twist your forearm as you go down and you will also exercise your triceps.

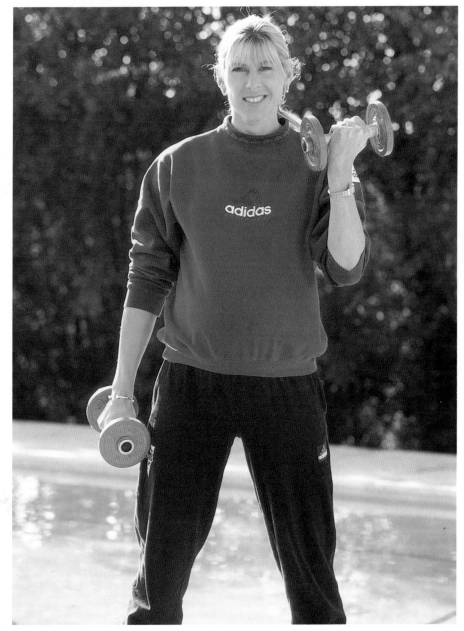

2. DUMB-BELL PUNCH

This should be a smooth and controlled exercise, and your body should be still to gain the maximum benefit to your shoulders. Note that my sweatshirt is not designed to cover a big belly!

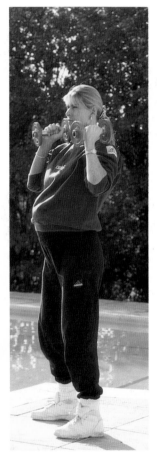

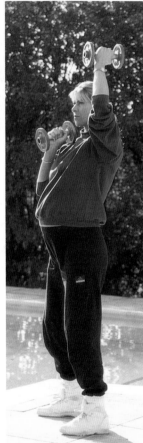

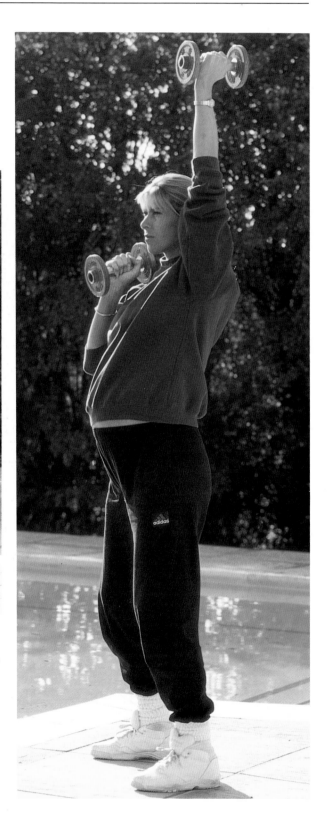

Stand with your feet apart, knees slightly bent, bottom tucked in. Hold the dumb-bells at shoulder height. Slowly straighten your arms *upwards one at a time - you should feel your shoulder muscles squeeze as you do this. Repeat 10 times on each side.*

3. SIDE RAISES

As well as working the muscles of your neck and across your shoulders, this exercise also uses your pectorals. Keep your elbows soft.

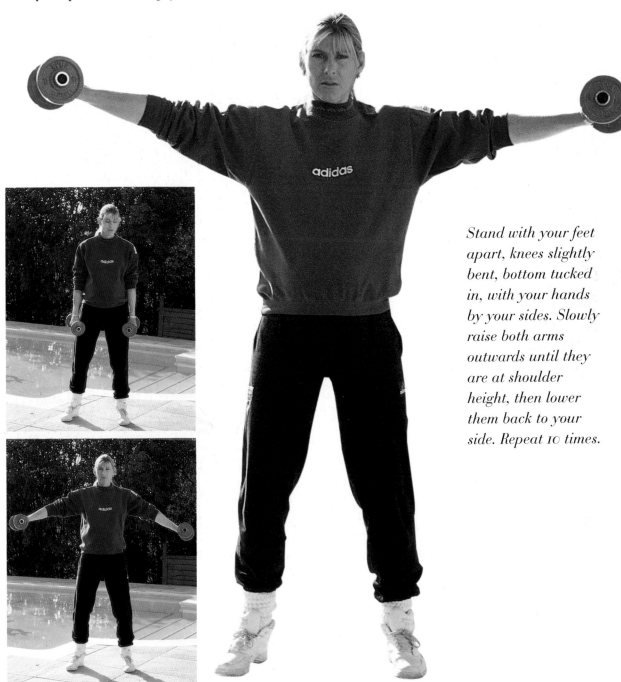

Stand with your feet apart, knees slightly bent, bottom tucked in, with your hands by your sides. Slowly raise both arms outwards until they are at shoulder height, then lower them back to your side. Repeat 10 times.

BACK ARCH

This is a wonderful stretch that uses the muscles in your bottom and the back of your legs, and helps to keep your back supple. Don't use your shoulder muscles to lift yourself off the ground.

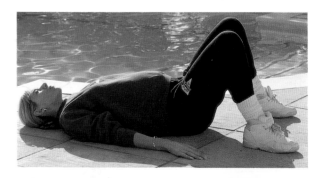

Lie on your back, with your knees bent and your feet flat. Keeping your shoulders on the floor, gradually lift your bottom off the ground, then lower it down again.

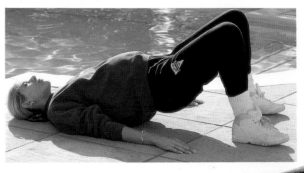

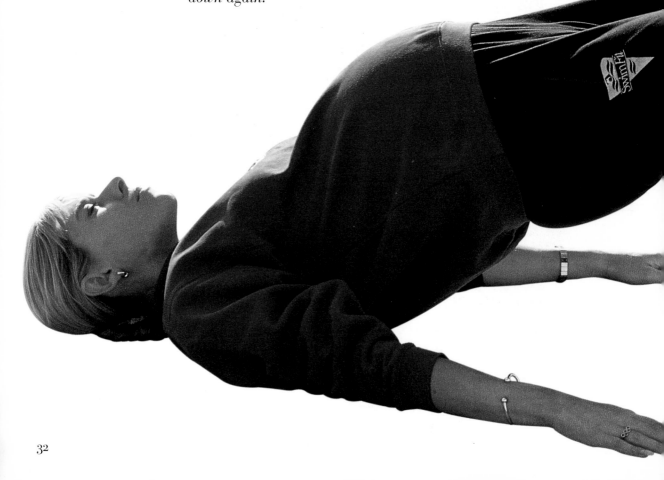

To extend this exercise further you can twist your knees and hips first to one side then the other, but don't strain. Beware if you have lower back problems.

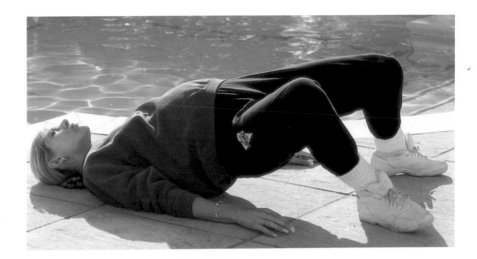

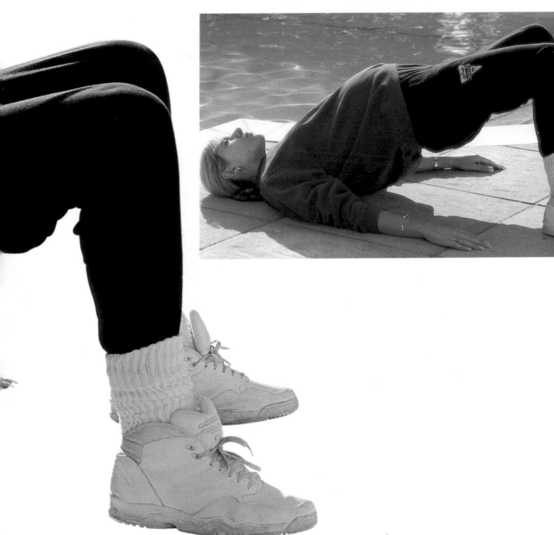

SIDE STRETCHES

There is no need to go too far with this exercise. What is important is that you are aware of the muscles working in your sides as you bend.

Stand straight with your bottom tucked in, knees slightly bent, and place your hands either on your hips or supporting your lower back. Slowly bend to one side, return to the middle then stretch the other way. Repeat 10 times on each side.

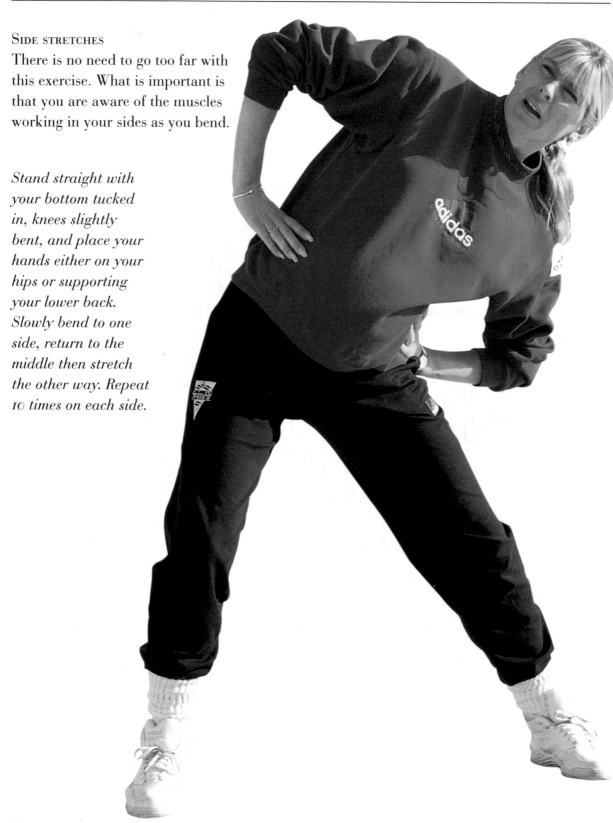

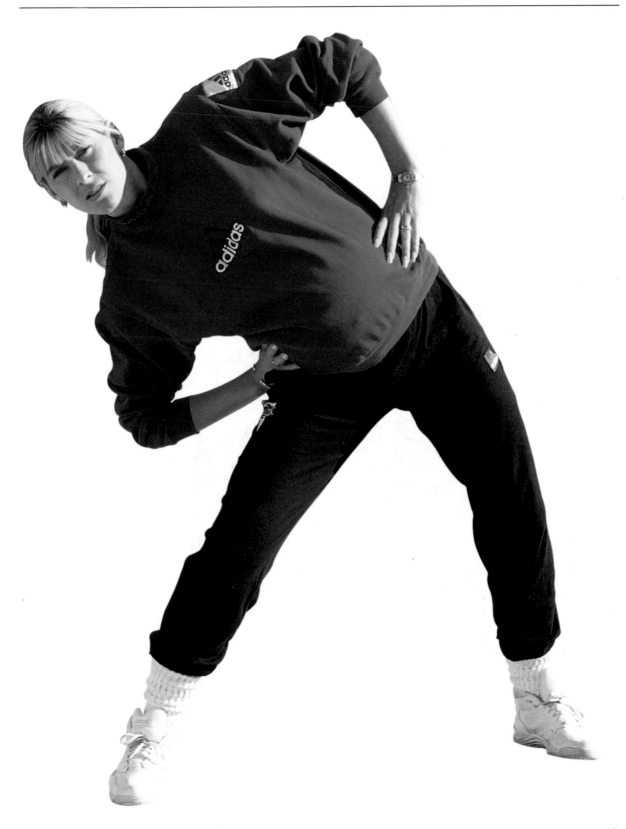

CONTROLLED LUNGE

When you are pregnant you can put your hands on your lower back for support while you do this exercise, and be careful not to lunge too enthusiastically or you may not be able to get back up again. This works the front of your back leg and the back of your front leg. When you are not pregnant you can do this exercise with a weight in each hand, and can increase the length of your step.

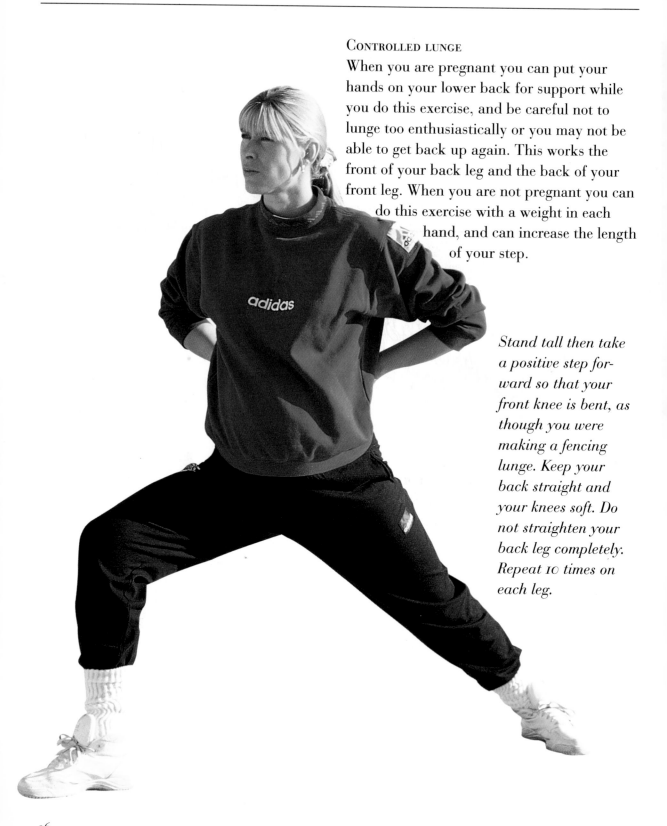

Stand tall then take a positive step forward so that your front knee is bent, as though you were making a fencing lunge. Keep your back straight and your knees soft. Do not straighten your back leg completely. Repeat 10 times on each leg.

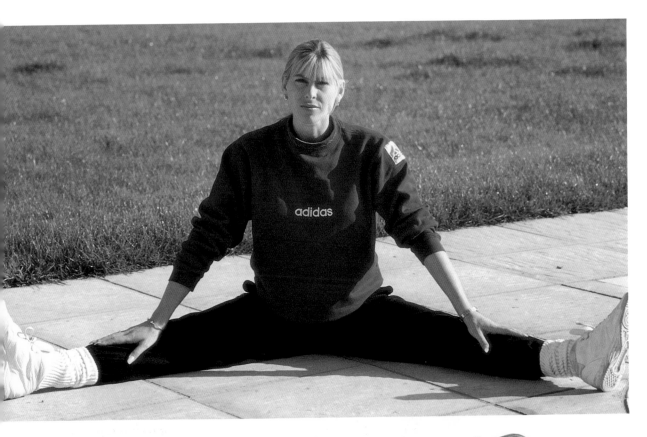

SEATED SIDE STRETCH

This should be a smooth stretch, not an abrupt movement. Sit tall and stretch from your tum and the bottom of your back, and lead with your nose, not the top of your head.

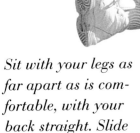

Sit with your legs as far apart as is comfortable, with your back straight. Slide your hands towards

your ankle until you feel a stretch and hold as long as possible. Return to the central position

then repeat on the other side. If you prefer you can place your hands on the floor on either side

of your leg to support your weight. Repeat three or four times on each side.

Cat stretch

A cat always has a good stretch when it first wakes up, and we should do the same. Because your spine relaxes while you sleep you are actually slightly taller when you first wake up, but during the day your vertebrae become compressed. This stretch gives you a wonderful relaxed feeling and will keep your back supple.

Kneel on all fours. Drop your stomach and pull up your shoulders and bottom, then reverse the position so that your back is arched and your shoulders and bottom are down. Repeat eight to 10 times.

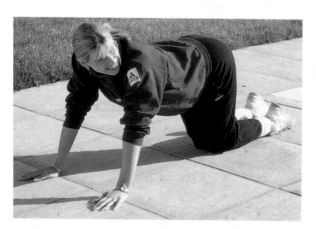

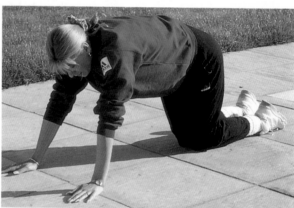

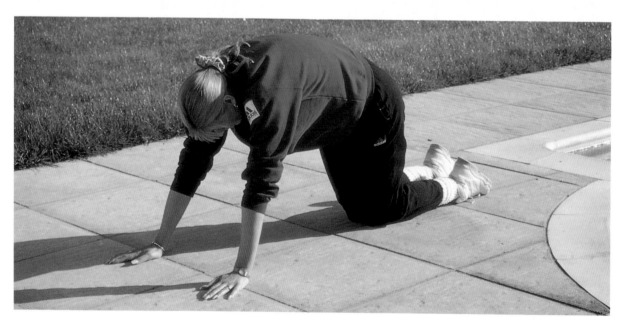

UPRIGHT BENT KNEE LEG RAISE

Make sure that the chair you use for support will not tip over. This exercise works the top of the thigh muscles (called your hip flexors). Don't worry if you can't lift your leg very high. Just do what you can without losing your balance or over-straining. Make sure this is a controlled squeeze. There is less benefit if you do it quickly, and you are more likely to over-balance.

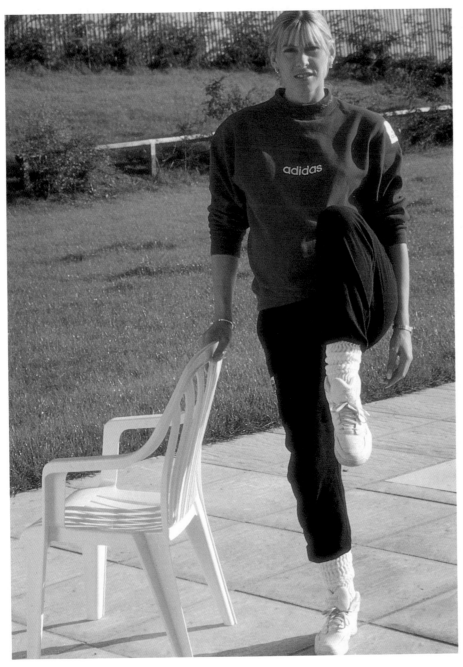

Stand straight, but keep your knees soft. Raise your leg with your knee bent then put it down again. Repeat 10 times each side.

CALF STRETCH

This is a very simple but effective exercise. Again, make sure that your chair is secure. Keep your supporting leg slightly bent.

Stand with one foot in front of the other. Then keeping your heels on the ground slowly bend your knees to feel a stretch on the calf muscles of your back leg. Repeat eight to 10 times.

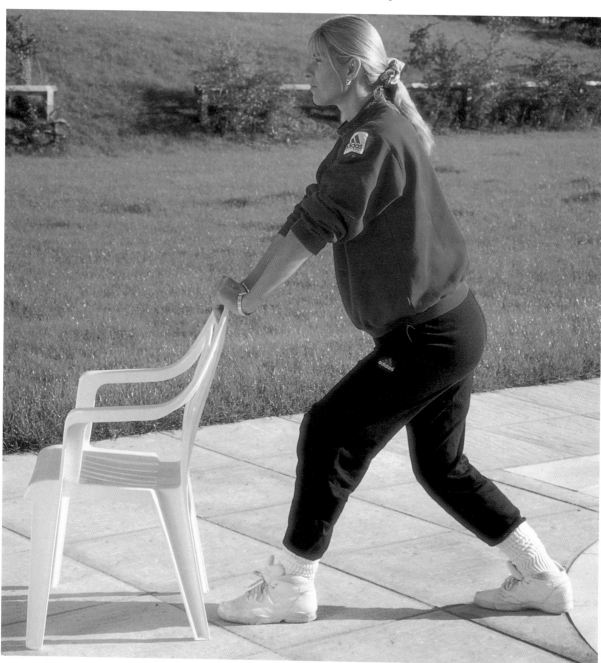

BOTTOM STRETCH

This is another exercise which is simple to do and yet gives a good stretch to the muscles in your bottom.

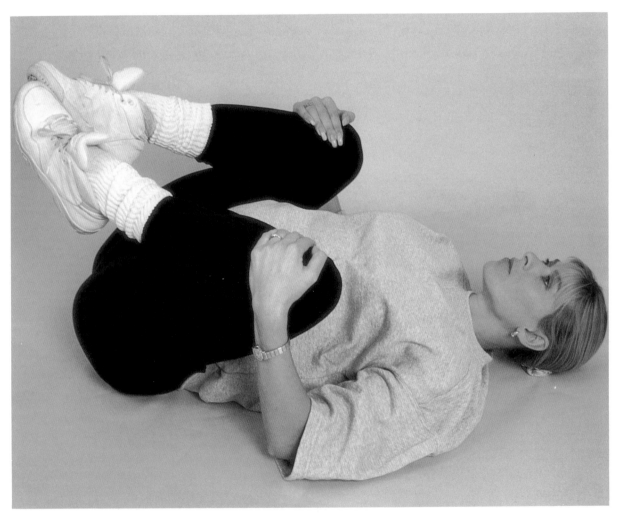

Lie on your back then pull up your knees towards your chest. (You will need to put them either side of your bump.)

Squeeze and release five to 10 times to feel a stretch.

BACK ARCHES

These two exercises are complementary. You may not be able to do them in the later stages of your pregnancy, and you should also avoid them if you have any back problems. Both stretch your lower back and neck. This is the part of your back which aches during pregnancy and this exercise may help to relieve it.

a) Supporting your weight on your arms so that your bump is off the floor, lie on the front of your legs.

Gradually turn to look over one shoulder, then turn to look over the other. Repeat five times on each side.

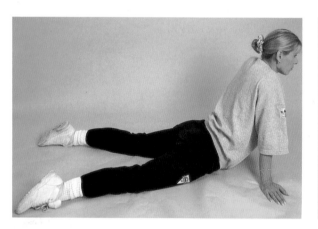
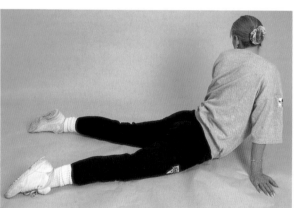

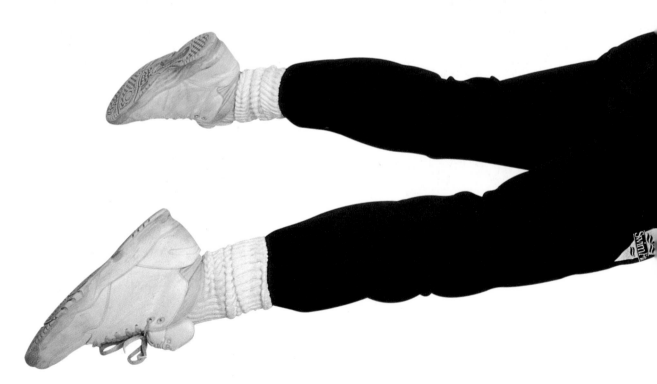

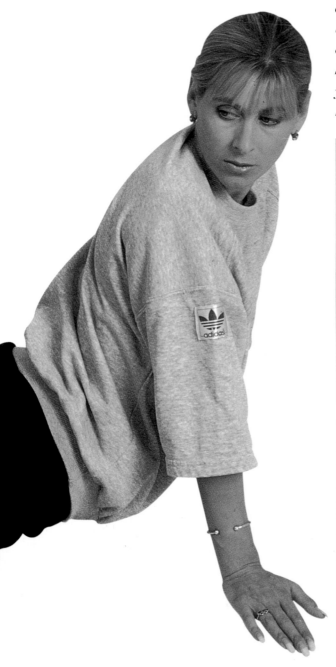

b) Support your hips on your hands and bring your legs up and over your head. Straighten them if you can and get as near to the floor as is comfortable. If you manage this, you can then extend this exercise by walking your toes first to one side then to the other.

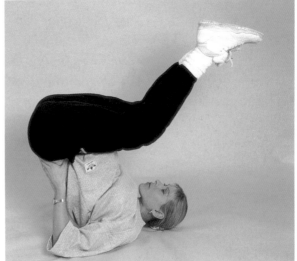

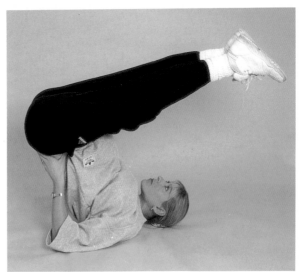

HIP FLEXORS

The important point with this exercise is not to arch your back, but to concentrate on loosening your hips and stretching your thighs.

Lie on your back with your knees bent and rest your hands lightly on your tummy. Starting with your feet as flat you can get them, rock your knees first to the left, then to the right. Repeat 10 times on each side.

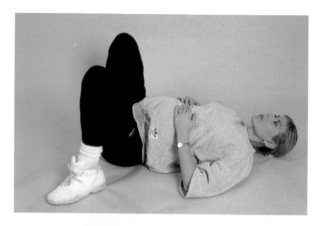

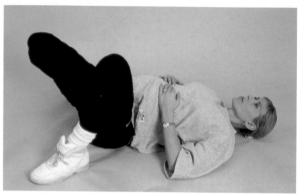

THIGH SQUEEZE

This exercise should be done smoothly, as with all the exercises, and will tone up your inner thighs.

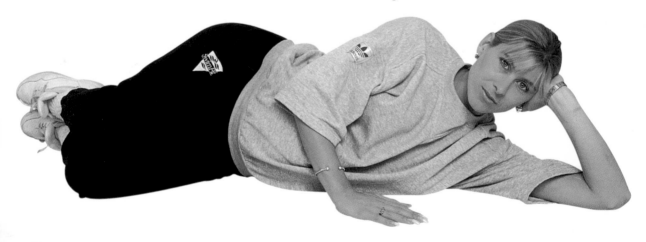

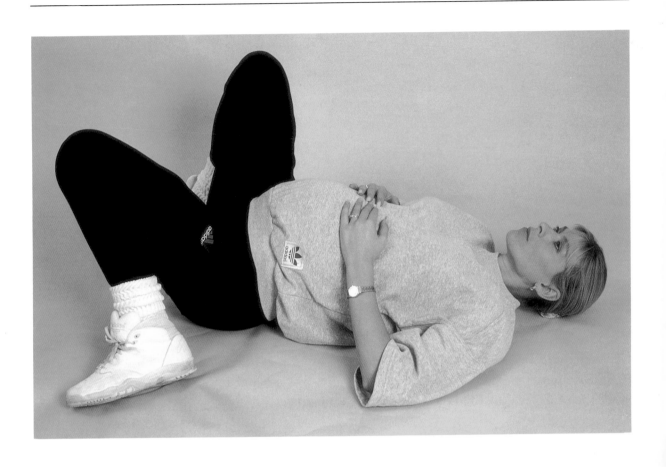

Lie on one side with your knees bent and your feet together, *and lean up on your lower arm. Gently raise and lower the* *upper leg without twisting your hip and feel the muscles in* *your inner thigh working. Repeat 10 times on each side.*

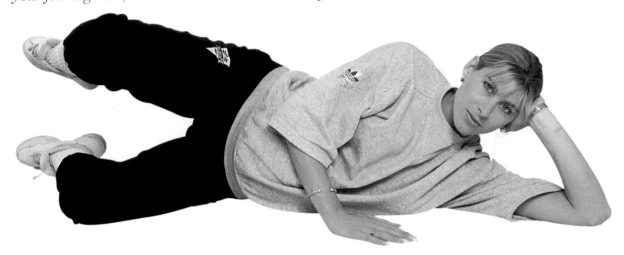

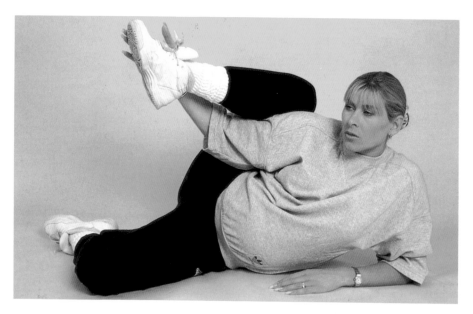

BOTTOM AND HAMSTRING FLEX

OK so perhaps I was more supple than some pregnant mums, so don't be discouraged if you cannot achieve the final position in this sequence. Just go as far as you can. This exercise is in two parts, and the first half works on your bottom, the second on your hamstring.

Lie on your left side with your left leg bent and lean up on your left arm. Wrap your right arm around your right leg. Move your right foot in towards your chest then back to the original position.

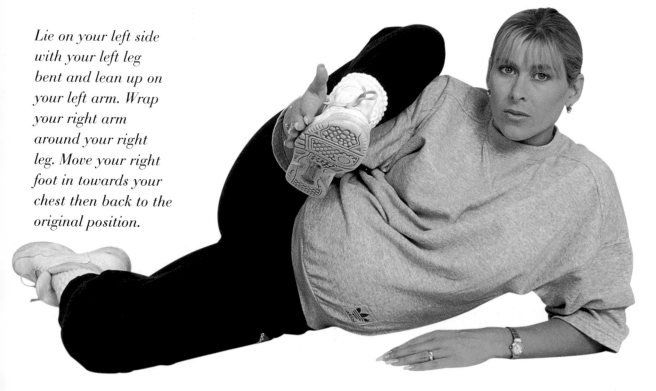

From the same starting position, extend your leg vertically as far as you can. Then bend your knee again. Repeat five times on each side.

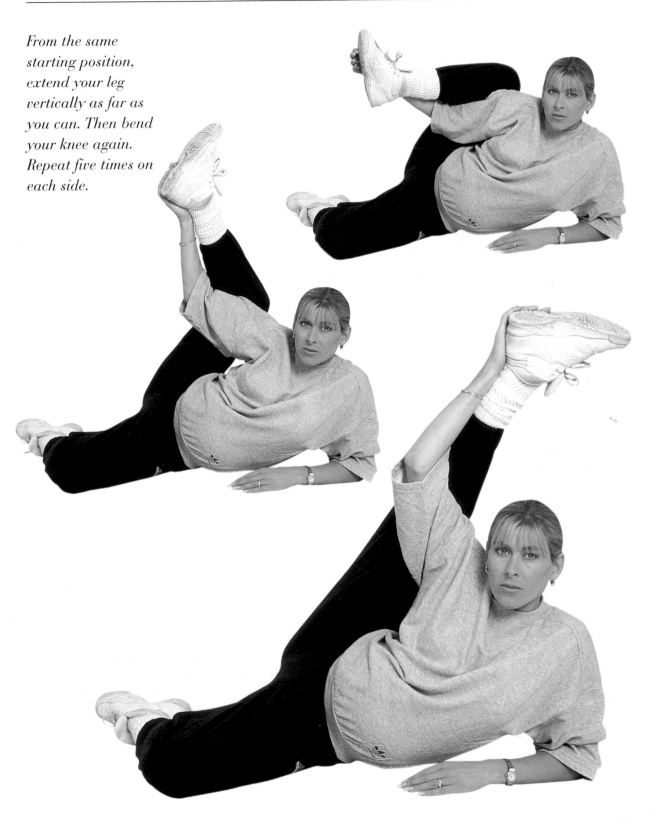

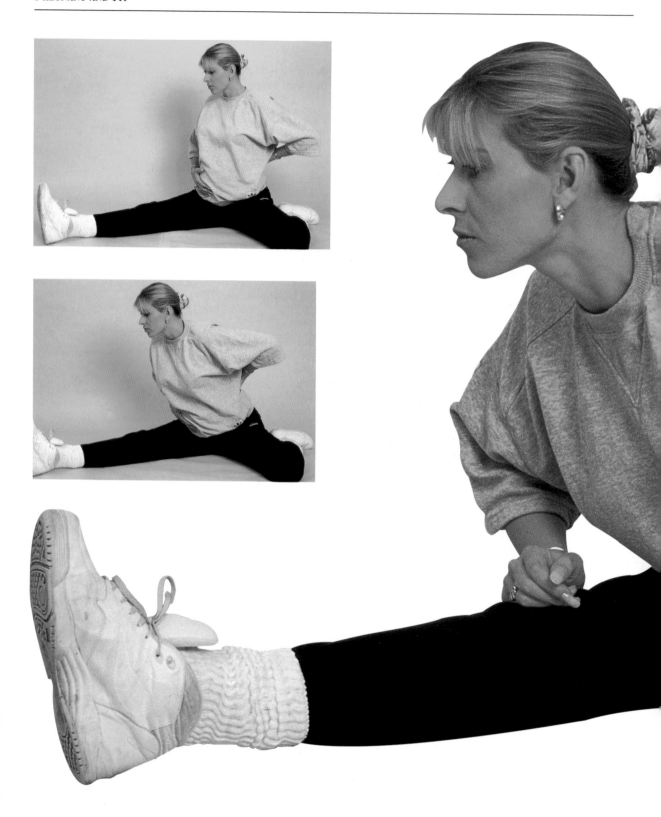

HURDLE STRETCH

This routine is designed to stretch your hamstring and the muscles in your lower back. Be aware of your bump and retain good posture. The idea of this exercise is *not* to put your nose on your knee! It should not hurt but you should feel a gentle stretch.

Sit in classic hurdle position, that is, sit upright with your right leg out in front of you, toes pointing to the ceiling, and bend your left leg 90° (or as close as you can manage) with your foot behind. Support your bump with one hand, and place the other hand in the small of your back. Gently and without jarring, sit tall then lean forwards as though trying to see what is beyond your toes. Gently lean as far forward as your bump will allow, without straining your back. Use your right arm to support yourself if you need to, then slowly and smoothly sit up again. Repeat three to five times on each side.

DYNA-BAND EXERCISES

The Dyna-band shown here is available from most good sports shops for about £8, and is an excellent investment. It can be tightened or loosened depending on whether you want to work hard or take things a little easier and you should not have it so tight that it flips out of your hands or you will hurt yourself.

1. PECTORAL STRETCH

As well as toning your pectoral muscles in your chest, this exercise will also firm up your underarms and tone your shoulders.

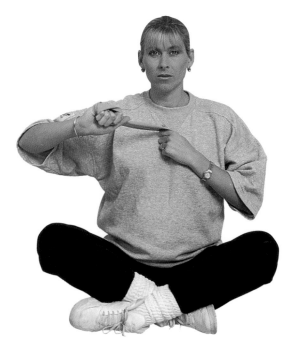

Sit comfortably, with your back straight and not arched. Hold the band firmly in both hands at shoulder height. Slowly and smoothly straighten your right arm, keeping your hands at shoulder height. Controlling the band, release the tension and return to the starting position. Repeat 15 to 20 times on each side, increasing the tension as you improve.

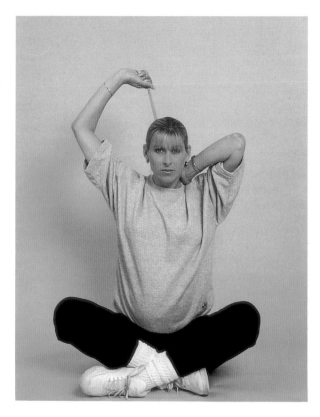

Vary this stretch by pulling the band up and back behind your head.

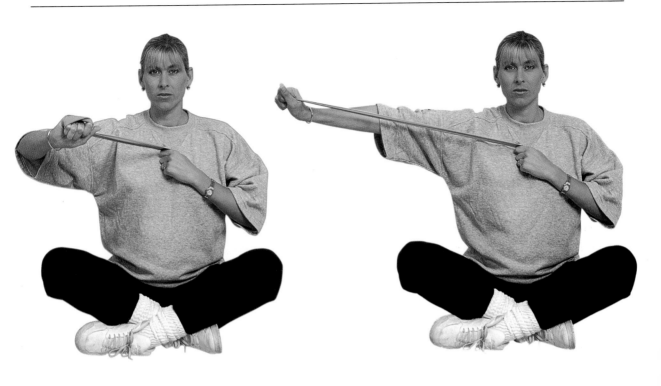

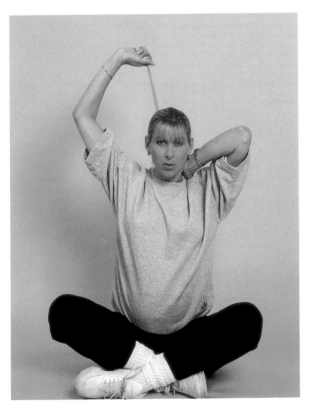

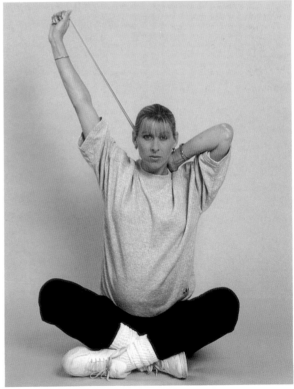

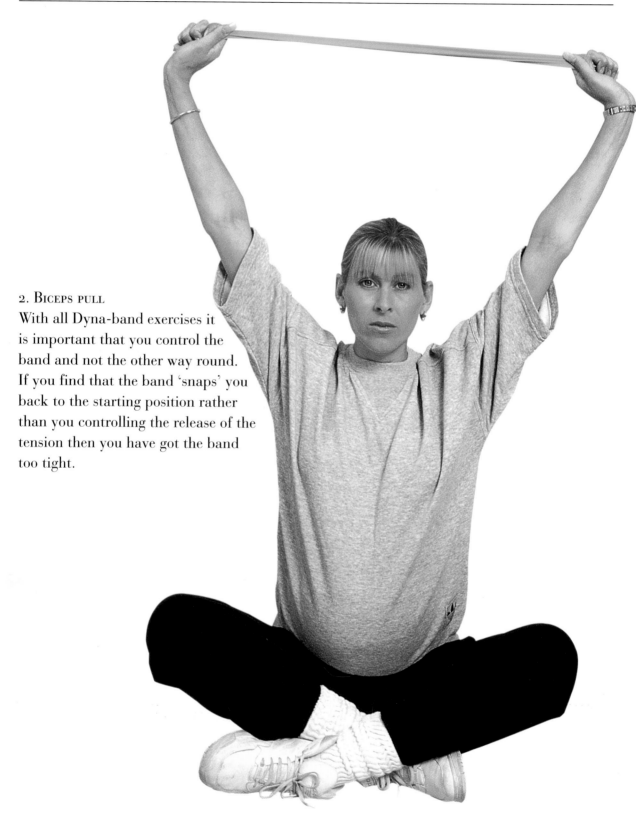

2. BICEPS PULL

With all Dyna-band exercises it
is important that you control the
band and not the other way round.
If you find that the band 'snaps' you
back to the starting position rather
than you controlling the release of the
tension then you have got the band
too tight.

Sit with your legs crossed and your back straight. Put your arms above your head and stretch the band out and down. Slowly release the stretch then lower your hands to shoulder height and repeat the stretch behind your head. Stretch 10 times in each position. Keep your elbows soft.

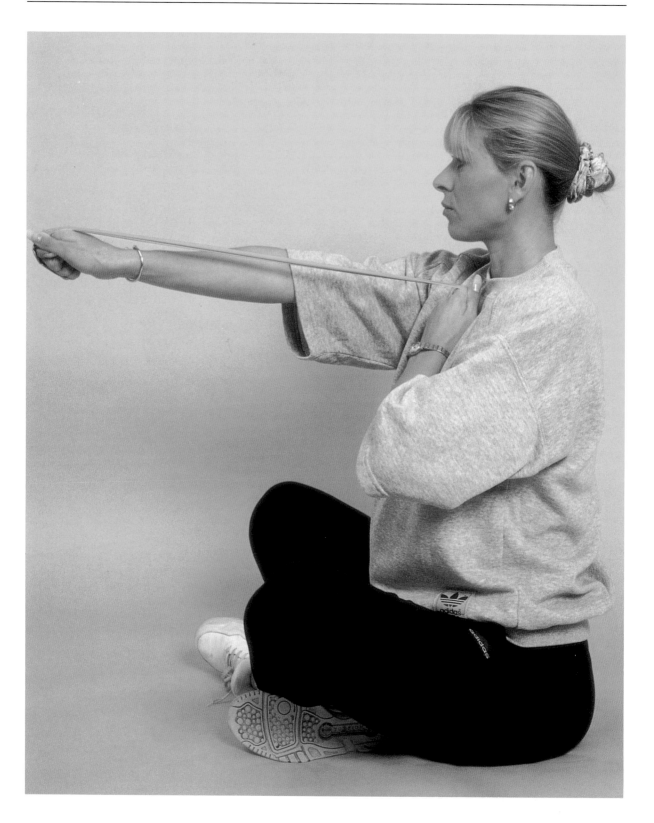

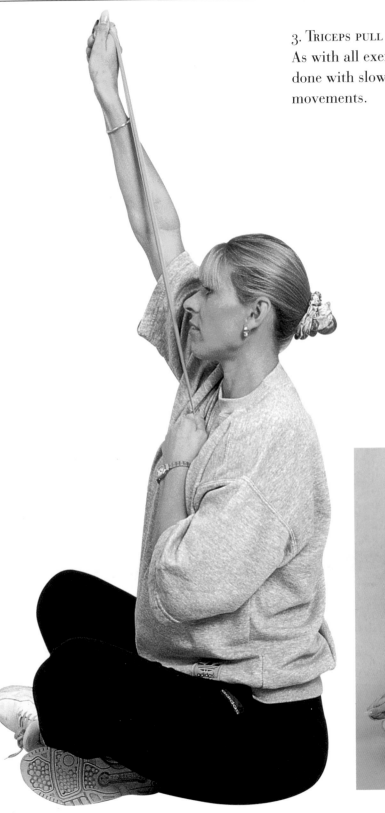

3. TRICEPS PULL

As with all exerices, this stretch should be done with slow, strong squeezes not abrupt movements.

Sit comfortably and hold the band securely. Keep one hand in at your chest and extend the other out in front to a count of three, and back, above your head, and back, then down towards the floor, and back. Repeat whole sequence eight to 10 times on each side.

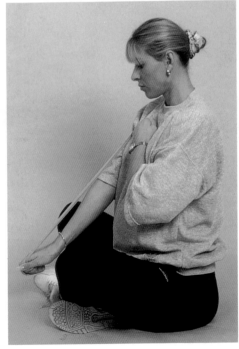

4. DOUBLE TRICEPS PULL

Make sure that the band is secure around your foot. For a variation on this exercise you can wrap it around both feet.

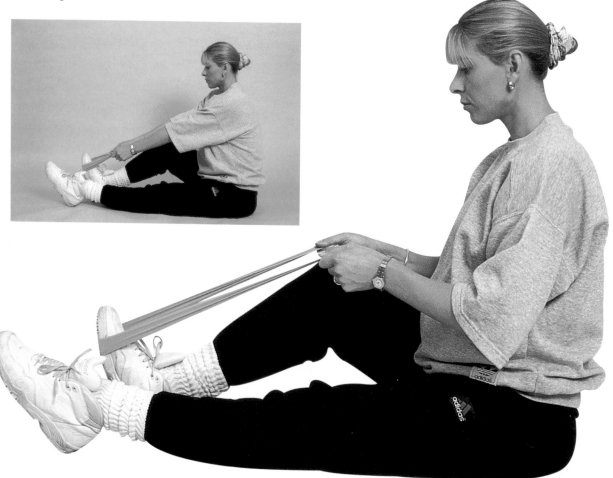

Sit straight with your legs out in front of you. Bend one knee slightly and wrap the band around the foot of that leg.

Using both hands, pull the band towards you to a count of three, then control the release. Repeat 10-15 times.

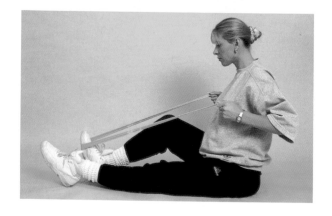

5. INNER THIGH PULLS

Towards the end of your pregnancy you might find that your bump is too big for you to do this exercise easily.

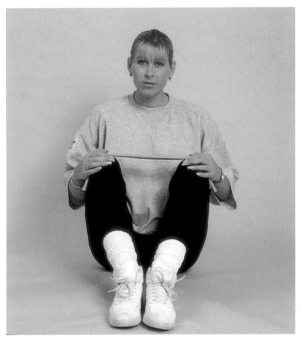

Sit comfortably and hold the band across your bent knees. Pull your knees apart against the band, and control the release of the tension back to the starting position. Repeat 10-15 times.

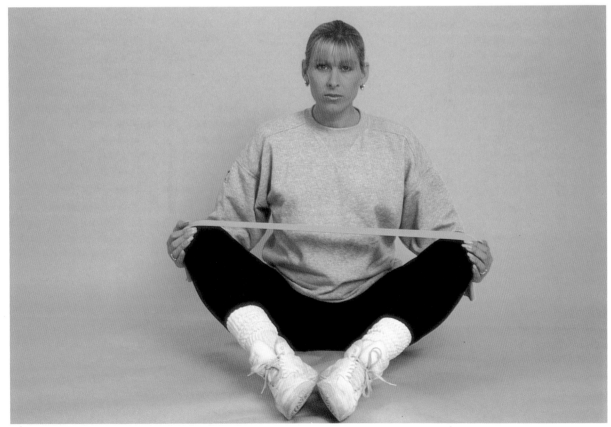

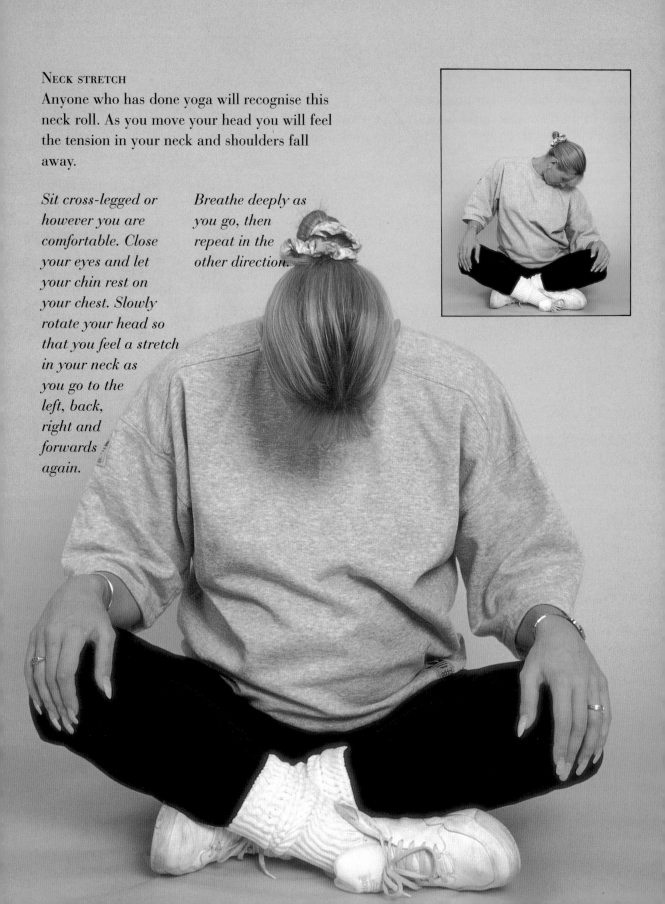

NECK STRETCH

Anyone who has done yoga will recognise this neck roll. As you move your head you will feel the tension in your neck and shoulders fall away.

Sit cross-legged or however you are comfortable. Close your eyes and let your chin rest on your chest. Slowly rotate your head so that you feel a stretch in your neck as you go to the left, back, right and forwards again.

Breathe deeply as you go, then repeat in the other direction.

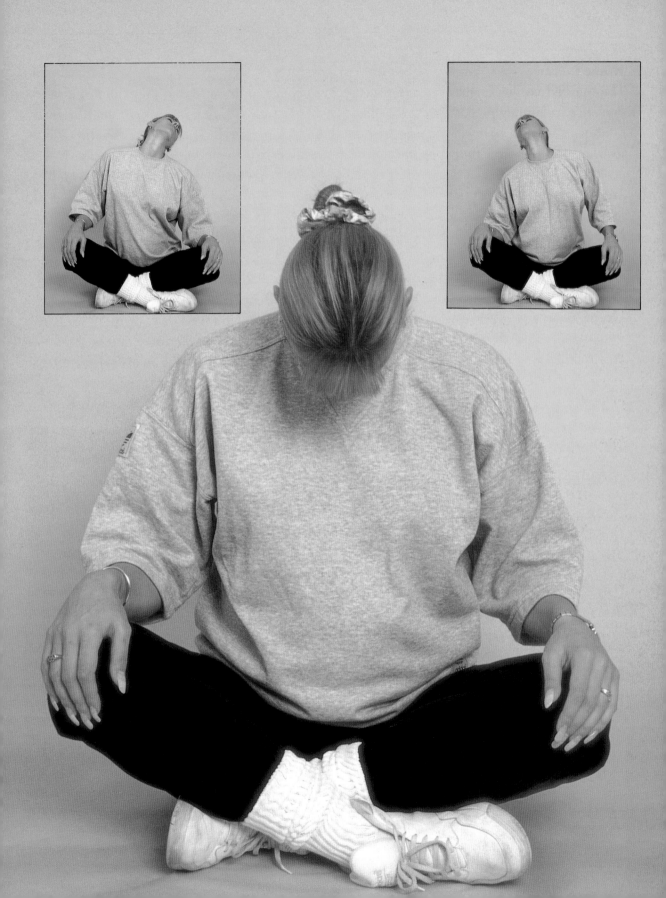

Water exercises

The wonderful thing about exercises that are done in a swimming pool is that the water takes your weight, while also offering good resistance that ensures that your muscles are given a good work-out. When you are heavily pregnant and feeling like a whale, it is lovely to lie in the water and move with grace and elegance again. Whatever gentle swimming you do, it doesn't matter if you don't use a correct swimming stroke. All exercise is good exercise, and an easy side stroke is just as acceptable as a perfectly executed front crawl.

Once you are in the water other swimmers might not be able to tell that you are pregnant. If you are swimming up and down in a lane it is worth alerting other swimmers to your condition so that they can be extra careful not to bump into you or inadvertently to kick you in the stomach. Try to choose sessions which are fairly quiet: you don't want an enthusiastic child jumping in and landing on top of you. Check at your local pool: it might be possible for you to join in at a mums and toddlers session at which things might be a little calmer.

You can buy maternity swimming costumes which are specially shaped to accommodate your bump. However, they are quite expensive, not very flattering and no good to you afterwards. I bought an ordinary Lycra suit a size bigger than my usual one which 'grew with me' and which I can still use.

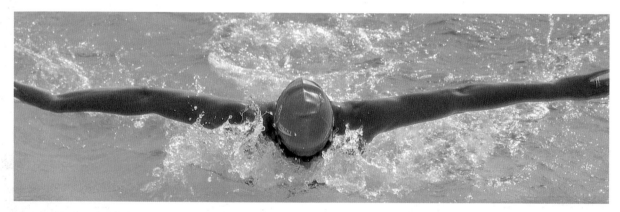

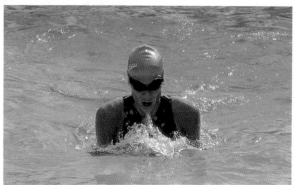

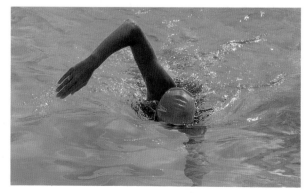

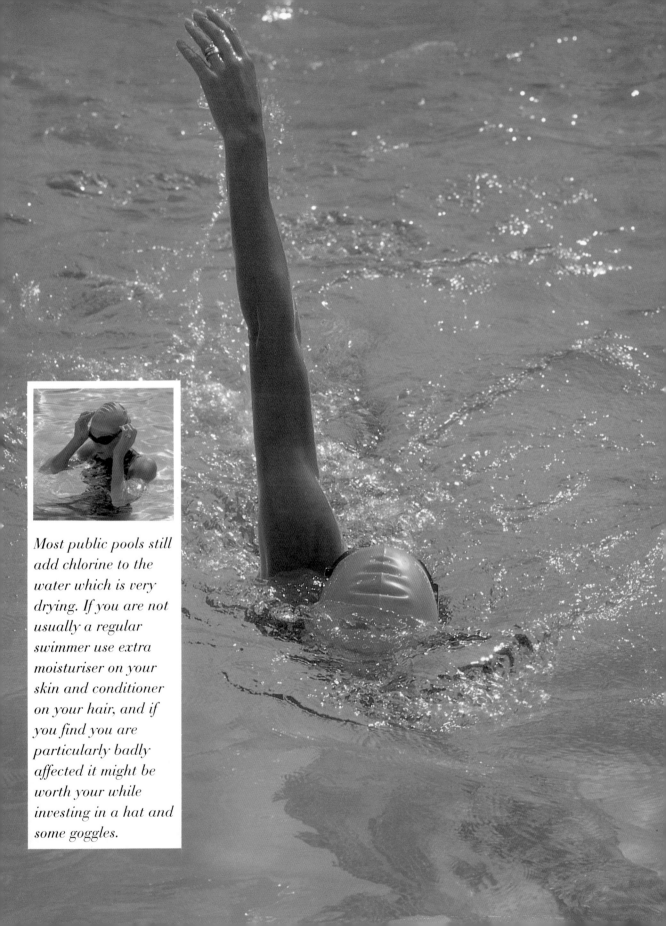

Most public pools still add chlorine to the water which is very drying. If you are not usually a regular swimmer use extra moisturiser on your skin and conditioner on your hair, and if you find you are particularly badly affected it might be worth your while investing in a hat and some goggles.

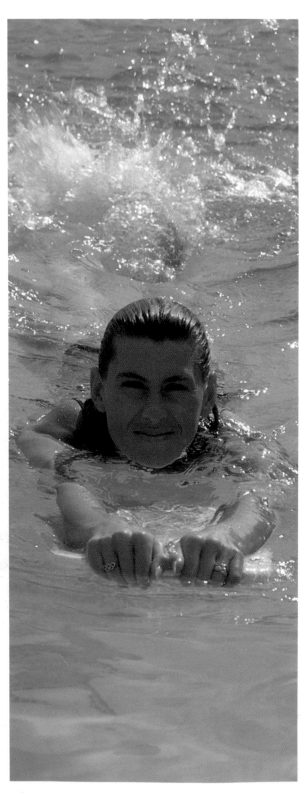

LEG KICKS

This exercise makes use of a float, which you can buy from good sports shops or which you might be able to borrow from your local swimming pool. How long you do this exercise will depend on how big you are and how quickly you get tired.

Lie on your front in the water and put the float in front of you with your arms outstretched. Kick your legs to propel yourself forwards.

Remember, don't bend your knees or make too much of a splash.

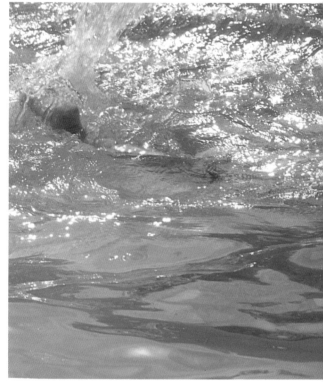

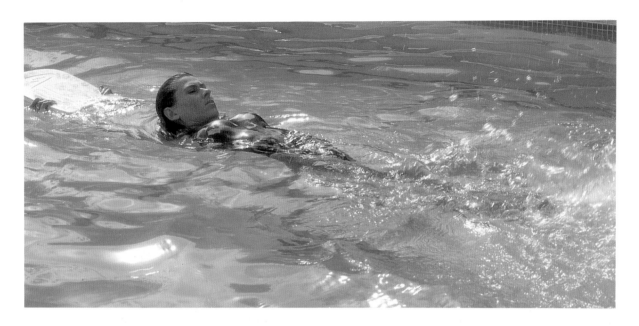

For a variation on this exercise, lie on your back and put your float behind you. Make sure your way is clear.

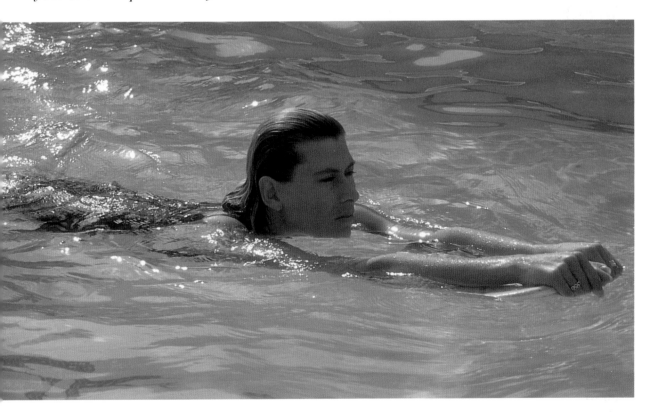

SCISSOR KICKS

Using the float helps you to stay on top of the water. This exercise works your bottom, legs and stomach.

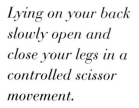

Lying on your back slowly open and close your legs in a controlled scissor movement.

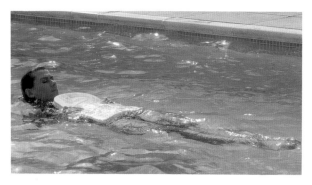

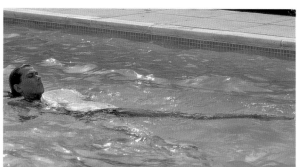

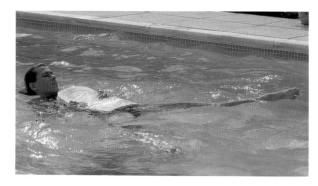

If your bump gets in the way put the float behind your head instead.

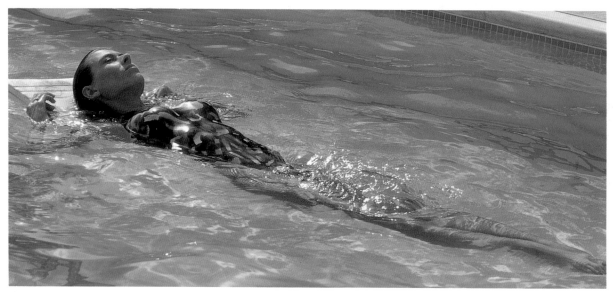

SCULLING

This simple exercise is good for your arms.

Still lying on your back and with your arms at your sides, gently scull your hands in the water.

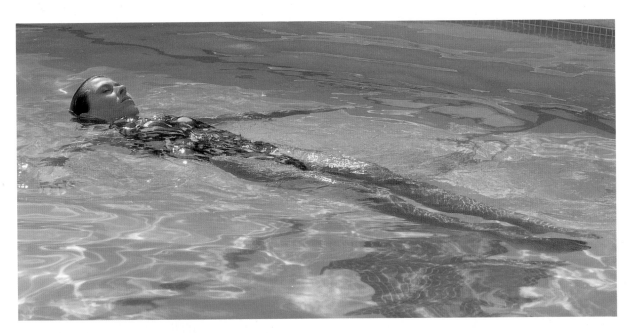

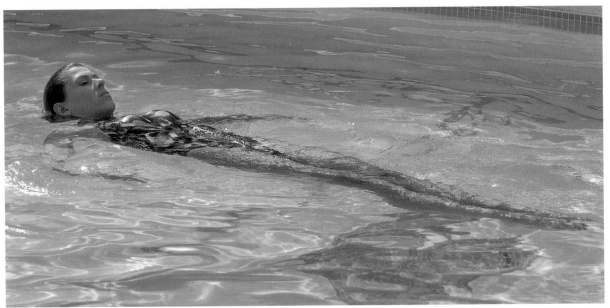

CONTROL POSITION

At the side of the pool hold on to the bar or trough, if there is one, or put one hand on top of the wall. Place your other hand flat on the wall under the water, with your fingers pointing downwards. This will keep you horizontal in the water.

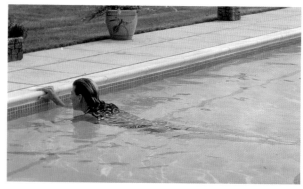

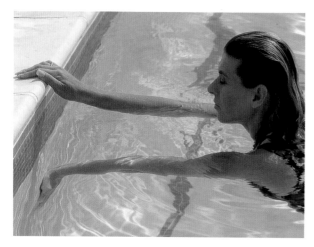

In this position, extend your legs behind you and repeat the scissor kicks described on page 64. Keep your body horizontal and make your movements slow and controlled. Repeat five to 10 times.

FLOAT PUSHES

Work your arms using the water as resistance.

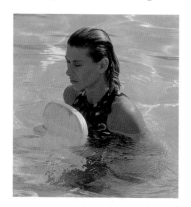
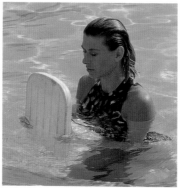
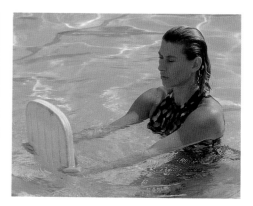

Squat or kneel in the pool and hold a float vertically half in and half out of the water.

Gently push and pull against the water. Repeat five to 10 times.

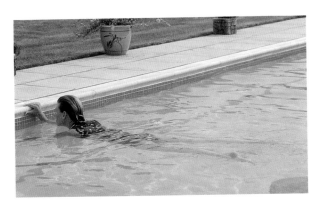

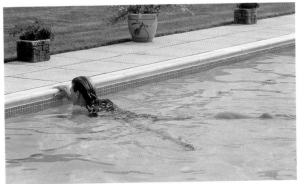

Now lie on your back sideways to the wall, still using one hand for support. Pull your knees in towards your chest and out again, up to 10 times. Make sure you change sides, because this exercise is quite hard on your supporting arm.

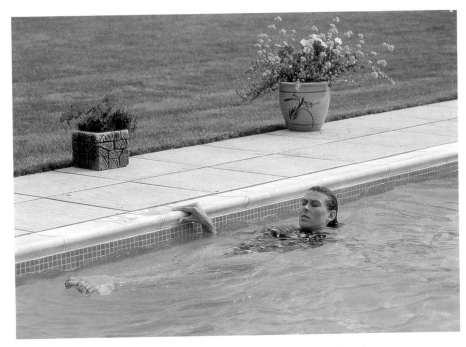

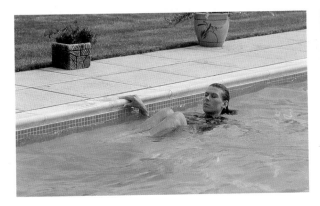

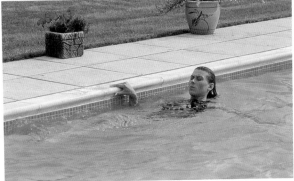

SWEEPS

This exercise is a good one if you are troubled by sciatica.

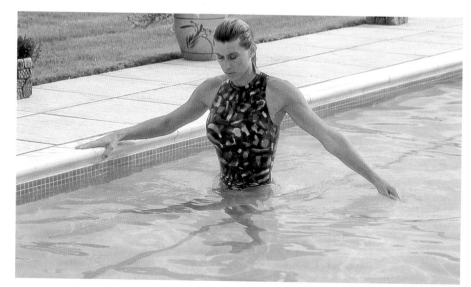

Hold on to the wall and sweep one leg across the other and back again. Repeat five to 10 times on each leg.

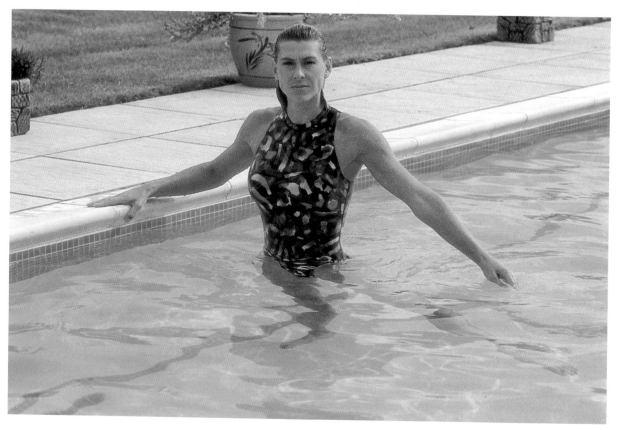

KNEE RAISES

This is an excellent work-out for your hipflexors.

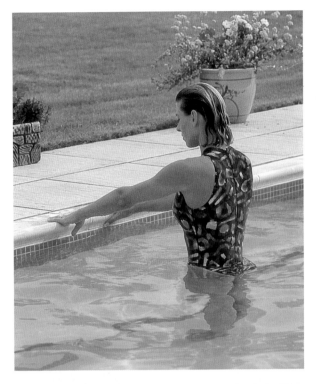

Stand facing the side of the pool and hold on with both hands. Slowly raise and lower your knee. Repeat five to 10 times on each side.

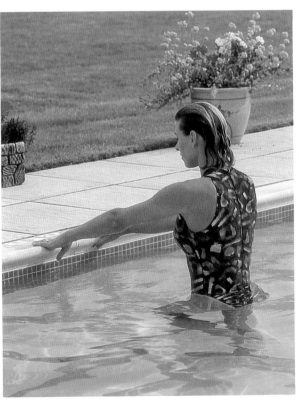

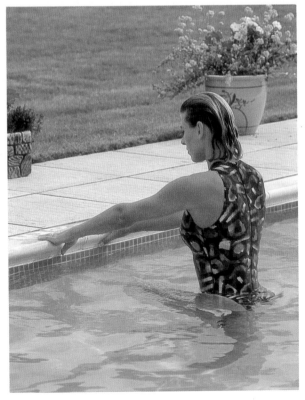

FROG MITTS

You can buy frog mitts from good sports shops or you might be able to borrow them from your local pool. If not, you can do this exercise by holding two small floats, or failing that just with the flat of your hand.

The mitts add extra resistance, and do the same for your hands as flippers do for your feet.

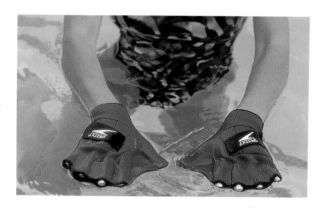

Sit so that the water is at shoulder height, then using the mitts (or floats, or your hands) squeeze your hands together with your palms inwards to work the inside of your arms . . .

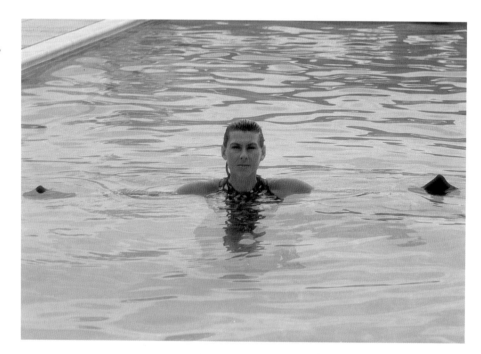

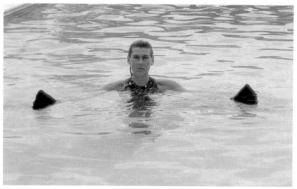

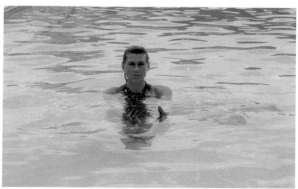

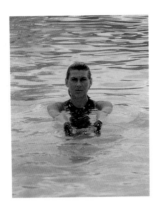

. . . then push them out with your palms facing outwards to work the outside of your arms.

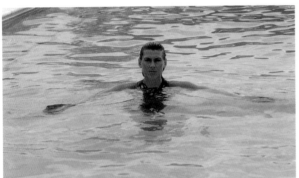

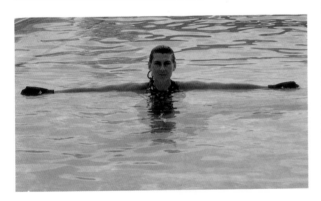

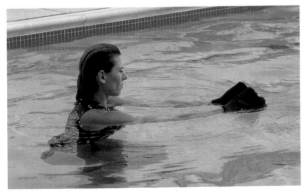

Pelvic floor exercises

If you don't do any other exercises for the whole of your pregnancy it is essential that you work your pelvic floor muscles. Actually we should all be doing this all the time, whether or not we are pregnant. The muscles between your pelvic bone and your coccyx support your internal abdominal organs and are the ones that take all the strain when you are delivering your baby, so you can see that you need to get them into good shape before the event and then work on them again afterwards to help them to recover. This is an exercise that you can do anywhere.

Pull in your muscles as if you were trying to stop yourself passing wind, and at the same time gripping a tampon and stopping the flow of urine. Relax and tighten 10-15 times in a row at least six times a day or as often as you remember. It is a good idea to associate it with some other activity, so that for instance every time you fill the kettle you also do this exercise.

Every time you go to the loo, try to stop the flow of urine and hold it for a count of 10, but make sure that you then empty your bladder properly afterwards.

You might not think that anything is happening when you first start to do this exercise, especially the first time you do it after your baby is born, but persevere because it is very important. (It is also good for your sex life!)

Chapter 5

MAINTAINING YOUR SELF-ESTEEM

I have already said that when you are pregnant your hormones play havoc with your emotions. At a time when everyone is expecting you to be 'blooming' and bursting with cheery anticipation it can be difficult to live up to this image. For much of the time you will feel fine, and happy, and full of the joys, but every now and then you will be thoroughly fed up of being pregnant – if not thoroughly fed up of everything.

The one thing you must keep telling yourself is that you are still a person inside that ever-expanding body, not just a 'baby-carrier'. Your partner can do wonders in this area if he is able to give you extra reassurance that he still thinks you are wonderful, so don't shut him out.

Of smocks and pinafores

To look at some of the maternity clothes that are available you would think that as soon as a woman becomes pregnant she loses all interest in fashion and has her sense of style mysteriously removed. Mercifully, however, some stores are now waking up to the fact that even mums-to-be want to keep on looking stylish and sexy, and there are one or two excellent mail order companies that specialise in trendy maternity clothes. You don't have to turn yourself into a frump for nine months.

There is no need to rush out and buy special clothes as soon as the test shows positive (unless you want to, of course). You will probably find that you can carry on wearing your normal clothes for several weeks until they start to feel too tight around the waist. The most important thing is to wear what you feel comfortable in. You could also have a rummage through your partner's wardrobe for larger t-shirts and sweatshirts, rather than spending a fortune on clothes that will be too small for the later stages of your pregnancy, but too big for you to wear when you return to your normal size. Stick to

It is possible to look sexy and stylish even when you are pregnant.

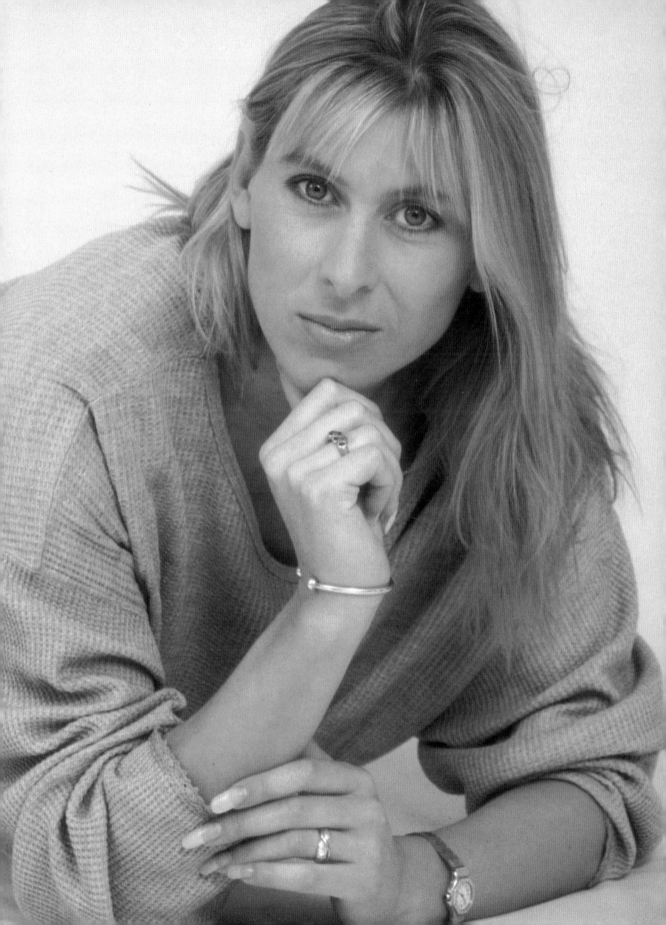

natural fibres where possible because you will feel warmer than normal. You can't look good if you feel sweaty and sticky. A good bra is important, too. You are likely to need a bigger size than usual fairly early on, and you will get even bigger before your baby is born. It is worth being properly measured if you are unsure of your new size. Drooping boobs are definitely *not* good for morale . . . If you are planning to breastfeed your baby will need to buy some proper nursing bras eventually, but don't bother until you are at least 36 weeks pregnant, after which time you are unlikely to get much bigger during your pregnancy although once your milk comes in you might get bigger still.

Leggings are a godsend. You can wear them anywhere and dress them up or down as required and they will carry you through all seasons, with long t-shirts in the summer and baggy sweaters in the winter. Don't forget, too, that if you have a special occasion to attend while you are pregnant you can hire outfits for a fraction of what you would have to pay if you were to buy something. And since you are unlikely to want to wear it again this makes good sense.

Don't be ashamed of being pregnant or feel that you have to withdraw from polite society until it is all over. Purpose-made maternity clothes might be comfortable, but there is no reason to put away your Lycra for a year. Some days I was happy to wear leggings and a baggy top, but equally on some days I wanted to wear something tight-fitting to show off my bump, so I did.

It is important to wear comfortable shoes. If you are used to teetering around on four-inch stilettoes you would probably feel rather strange in flatties. But if you don't want to end up with horrendous varicose veins and swollen ankles, try and be sensible about what you wear on your feet. Your legs will get more tired while you are pregnant and high heels will not help, and towards the end you will also find that your sense of balance is not all it should be, so be careful. Even so, if you are dressed up in your finery for a night out, no one would expect you to complement the outfit with a pair of trainers, so a low heel would be fine. If you find that your legs get very tired and your job means that you have to stand for long periods, invest in some support stockings. These are not as horrific as they sound, and in fact look just like ordinary tights: you won't look like Nora Batty!

Being pregnant does not mean you have to look dowdy.

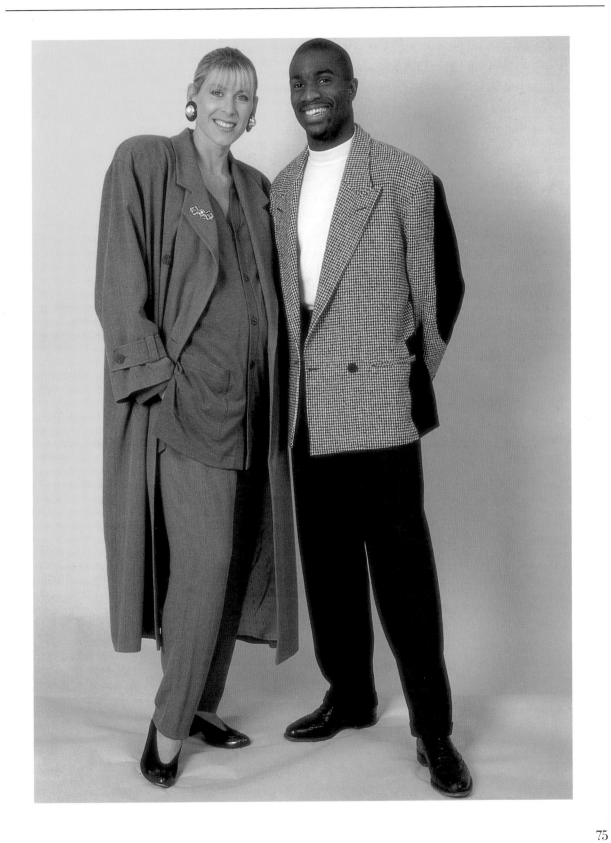

Hair today . . .

When I was expecting Elliott I had the sudden urge to change my appearance. I didn't want to have my hair cut because I thought that it was rather a drastic step, and one I couldn't go back on if I did not like the result. So instead I dyed my hair, and it went a reddish-orange colour which was certainly a change from my normal blonde but one I was quite pleased with for a while.

It is not a good idea to go for a completely new image when you are pregnant, because the chances are you are not really yourself to start with. It is best to avoid anything you are not sure about. Also, drastic chemical treatments such as perms or bleaches are probably not a good idea. However, a good hair trim will cheer you up, and it is lovely just to sit back and be pampered for a while.

Having a facial is another lovely way to spend an hour or so, too. In a similar vein it is worth checking where you live to see if any beauty counters are offering a make-over service. This is a surefire way of making yourself look wonderful, and again it is lovely to have some-one make a fuss of you for a while. Not only that, it may even be free!

Skin care

One of the early symptoms of pregnancy is often a change in the condition of your skin. Later you may get the characteristic 'glow', but at first you might find you suffer from unwelcome spots and pimples as your hormones do their stuff and the balance of your skin changes. There is not a lot you can do about this really, although a good diet and scrupulous cleansing might help. Again, it is one of the unpleasant 'side-effects' that is worse in the early months and settles down as your pregnancy progresses. Some expectant women find their skin itches. Try applying a good-quality moisturiser, some baby lotion or, if the itching is really driving you mad, some calamine lotion. If it gets unbearable or if you get any soreness on your skin, talk to your GP or midwife.

You will no doubt be worrying about stretch marks. You can buy special antenatal creams which make all sorts of claims, but again I think if you are going to get them, you are going to get them no matter what you do if you have that sort of skin. Generally, however, the better care you take of your skin, the more kindly it will take to

Cheer yourself up with a beauty treatment. A change of hair colour did the trick for Sharron.

Photograph: Express Newspapers.

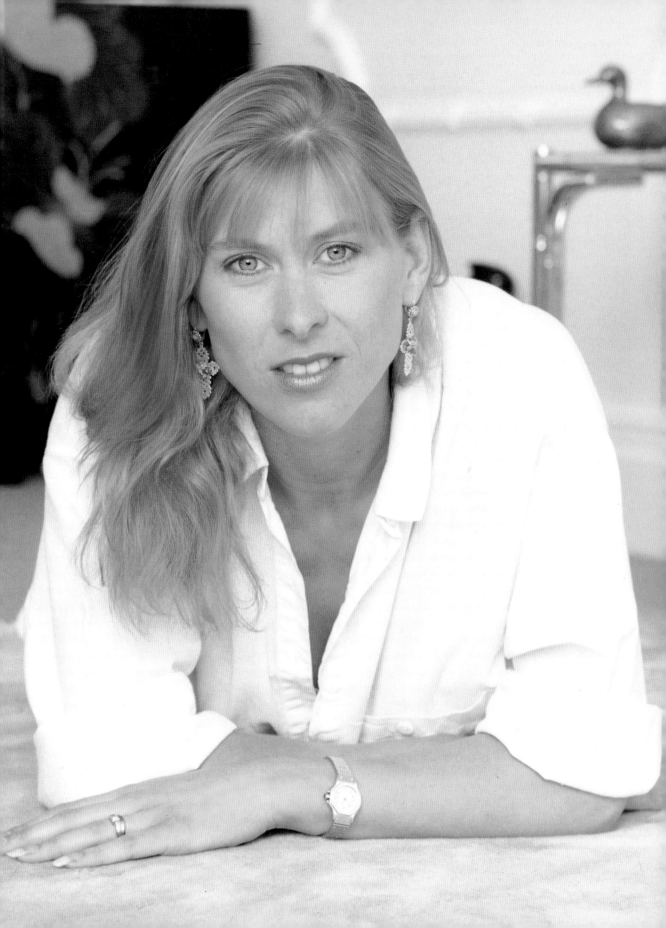

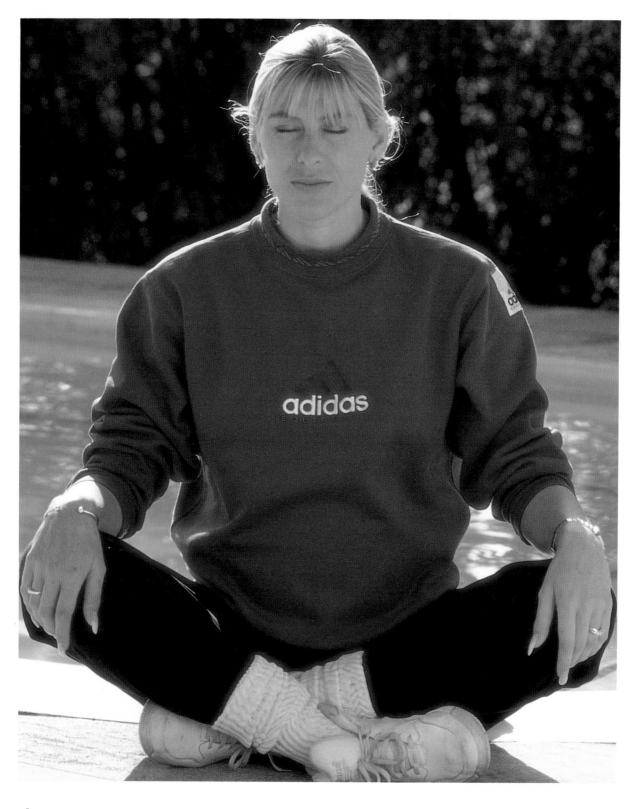

being stretched to its elastic limit, so keep smoothing on the moisturiser. Creams with vitamin E in them are particularly good, while gently massaging any marks which do appear might help them to vanish.

Another change in skin condition that some women experience is patches of darker pigment developing. This is only a temporary condition known as *chloasma* and is caused – you've guessed it – by the effect of your hormones, and will gradually disappear after your baby is born. Nipples also get darker, and a brown line appears on your abdomen which may not go away altogether.

Peace of mind

Try to put aside a little time each day just to sit for a moment and to try to relax. This is easier said than done if you are still working full-time and then coming home to look after older children and cook an evening meal. However, it is well worth the effort if you find even 10 minutes just to sit and ponder.

If you are attending antenatal classes you will be taught the importance of breathing properly, and how to relax. Sit or lie comfortably, close your eyes and try to relax all the muscles in your body. There are lots of different positions that are suitable for relaxing. Try sitting with your feet up in a chair that supports your back, lying on your back with pillows under your head, shoulders and thighs, or lying on your side with your upper leg bent and supported by a pillow: experiment until you find a position that is right for you.

Start at your toes and work your way up, tensing then relaxing your feet, legs, hips, stomach, arms and hands, shoulders, neck – even eyelids if you can – and as you do so try to visualise what your muscles are doing. Breathe slowly and deeply, pushing your stomach out as you inhale, then exhale slowly through your mouth. Try to empty your mind and just stay still and quiet for a little while. You might like to add some soothing background music if circumstances will allow. When you come up do so slowly, particularly if you have been lying down, or you will make yourself giddy and faint. Roll carefully on to your side, push yourself up on your arms, then stand up gently. It is amazing how good this can make you feel. Just ten minutes' relaxation can pick you up as well as an hour's nap.

Try to get some time aside just to calm yourself and practise some deep breathing.

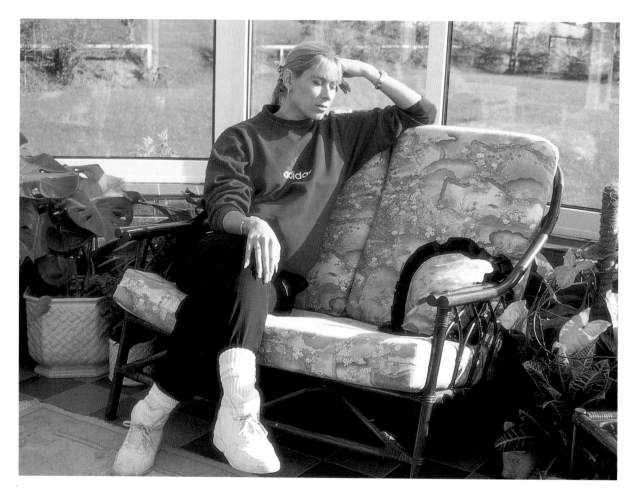

If you find that you start to feel stressed during the day but it's not convenient to lie down and breathe properly – if you are in a management meeting or pushing a trolley round the supermarket, for instance – take a few deep breaths, drop your shoulders, unclench your teeth, and give your arms and hands a shake. If you are sitting down, let your hands go limp and cup one inside the other with your palms upwards and breathe slowly and deeply.

Learn to relax and find time each day just to sit for a while.

Keeping sane

Just as it is important to keep up good habits as far as your physical well-being is concerned, so you should pay attention to your mental health. Part of the problem is that with the best will in the world people tend to focus on your baby and not on you, so unless you make some effort you might find yourself completely submerged.

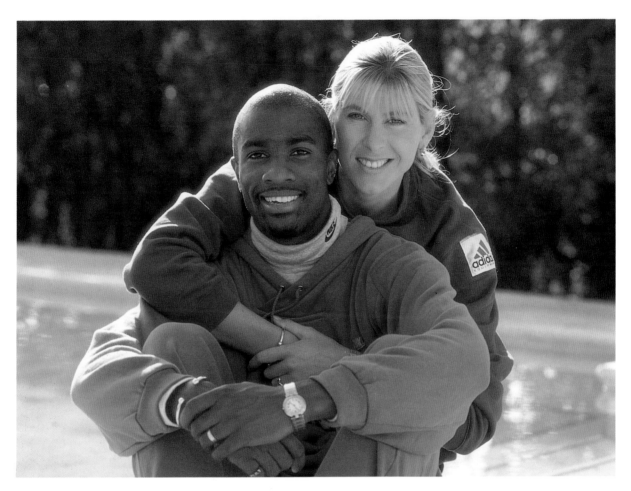

Make time to talk to your partner, to discuss any worries either of you has, and just to enjoy being together.

The advice for keeping physically fit can just as easily be applied to your mind. Start and maintain good habits now and you will find it easier to cope later. It is like climbing a mountain. Keep up slow and steady progress now, then if you do 'fall by the wayside' you will not have so far to catch up.

If you can, talk to other mums-to-be. You are bound to see them either at antenatal clinics or classes, or just as you go about your business. It is amazing how many you come across when you are one yourself. Years ago women had their own mums close at hand to talk to but if you do not live near your family you will have to set up your own support network. Even when everything is going smoothly it is nice to have someone to talk to who *really* knows how you feel at that moment. Don't be afraid to ask someone else's opinion if you have a nagging worry, no matter how silly you feel. The chances are that the

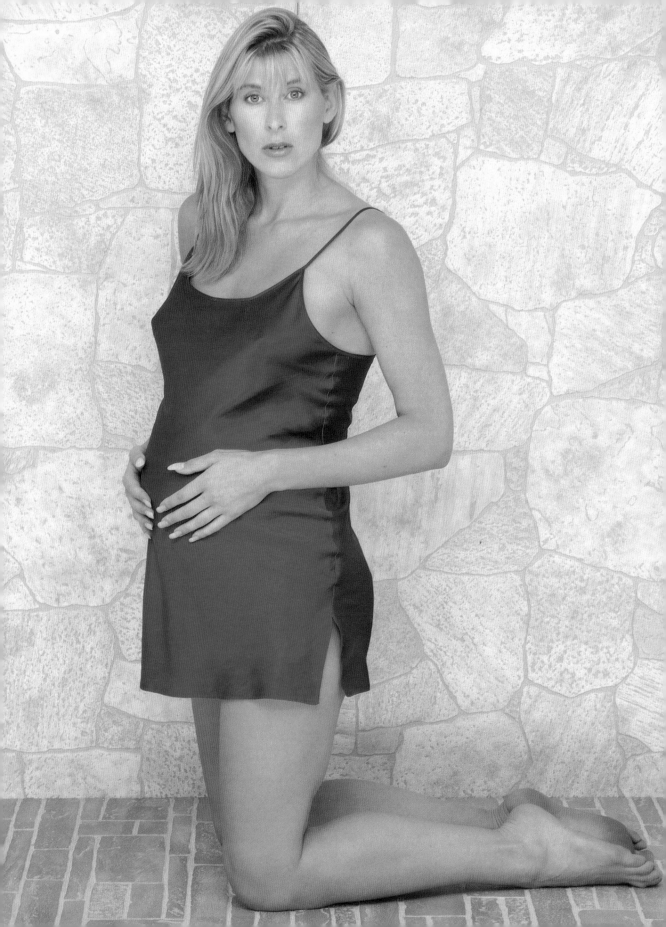

person you ask will have felt exactly the same at some point, and if you talk to a midwife or health visitor you can be sure that there is no question they haven't answered many times over. Make a note of any worries you want to mention at your next antenatal appointment because if you don't they will go clean out of your head. Even if your mum is on hand times have changed and what was current advice when you were born may not be in vogue today. Find out what the up-to-date information is and exchange ideas with other mums-to-be.

Talk to your partner, and explain how you are feeling – and don't forget to ask him how is he is today!

If you look good you will feel good, and your self-confidence will be high. Your mental fitness is as important as your physical well-being because your lifestyle is about to be turned upside-down and you need to be ready for this exciting challenge. As with physical exercise, you will have good days and bad days. Take advantage of your good days and try not to wallow on your bad days.

Eight and a half months pregnant – and still looking sexy.

Photograph: John Dietrich.

Chapter 6

USING YOUR TIME CONSTRUCTIVELY

The last few weeks of your pregnancy can seem very long. If you have recently given up work the sudden relative isolation can feel very strange, but there are lots of things you can do. If you have older children you won't need me to tell you that you will be very busy keeping up with the day-to-day routine of meals, washing, cleaning, etc, etc. On top of all this there are preparations to make and last-minute shopping to buy. If this is your first baby you might like to consider the following pointers on things that you need to do.

Look after yourself
Towards the end of your pregnancy you will be very tired so you might not feel like doing anything much, but take advantage of the last weeks of peace that you will have for quite a while. Do things that are just for you: visit an art gallery, go out to lunch with friends, take your partner to the theatre, finish that watercolour, read some good books.

Once your baby is born you will have little opportunity to take long, leisurely soaks in the bath, uninterrupted, so do it now. A warm, bubbly bath is a lovely pick-you-up, but when you have a persistent little voice demanding your attention it will be a luxury that you will not be able to indulge in as often as you might like.

Similarly you might like to have a last holiday as a couple, and if you are planning to go away, particularly towards the end of your pregnancy, there are a couple of sensible precautions you should take. Take your hospital notes with you, just in case, and check your insurance to make sure that maternity care is covered, especially if you are going abroad. If you want to fly check with your travel agent what the recommendations of the airline are. They might not let you fly if you are very pregnant, and in any event you are likely to need a letter

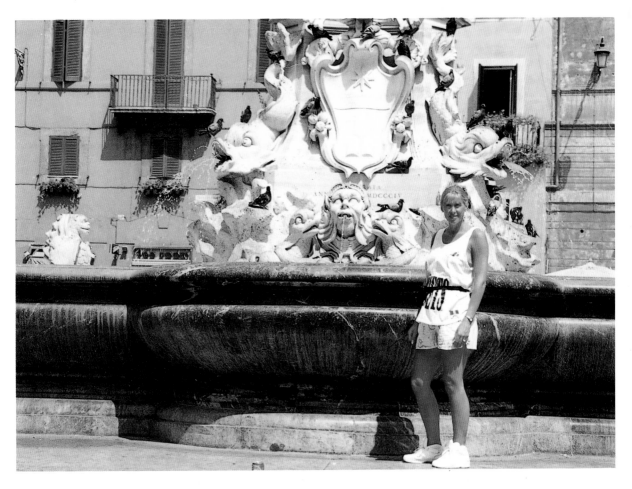

*On holiday in Rome,
six months pregnant.*

Photograph: Sharron Davies
collection.

from your doctor to confirm that he or she is happy for you to fly.
When I was six months pregnant we went to Rome by air, and I did
not have any problems. We had a wonderful time – including hiring a
motor scooter to travel around on, Derek, me and the bump!

If your budget will run to it, why not treat yourself to a beauty
treatment? Massage, aromatherapy, reflexology, a facial, a manicure
or pedicure are all good ways of being pampered and making you feel
good. This will boost your morale, if it needs it, and your confidence.
You won't be able to reach your toes by the end of your pregnancy, so
if you can get someone else to paint them for you that is wonderful. I
remember thinking as I lay in hospital with my legs split east to west
that I least my toenails looked good! It also got to be a struggle to put
on socks and shoes because my bump just got in the way.

If I had to give just one tip to an expectant mum I should say go to

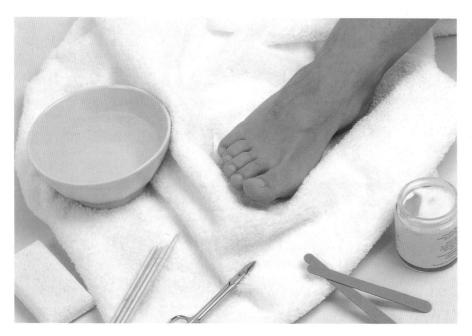

When you can't reach your feet any more, get someone to give you a pedicure.

bed for the last week of your pregnancy – you are going to need all the energy you can get!

Child care

If you are planning to return to work after your baby is born you will need to ensure that you have organised your child care arrangements.

If you are lucky your employer will run a creche, but the chances are that this will not be the case, so you will need to look elsewhere.

One of the most obvious choices is to ask a relative to help, perhaps grandma. On the face of it this is ideal, because you will be leaving your baby with someone that he or she already knows, and whom you know you can trust. However, think carefully about this: if you don't pay your mum (or whoever), as time goes on you might begin to feel beholden to them, or they might start to feel as though they are being taken for granted. But this is the very worst outcome, and most relatives are happy to help out. Even so, if your chosen carer starts to introduce something into your baby's routine that you don't entirely agree with, such as what he can eat, standards of behaviour and discipline, language and so on, it is easier to correct if you are instructing someone you are paying than it is to correct a relative who is, after all, doing you a favour.

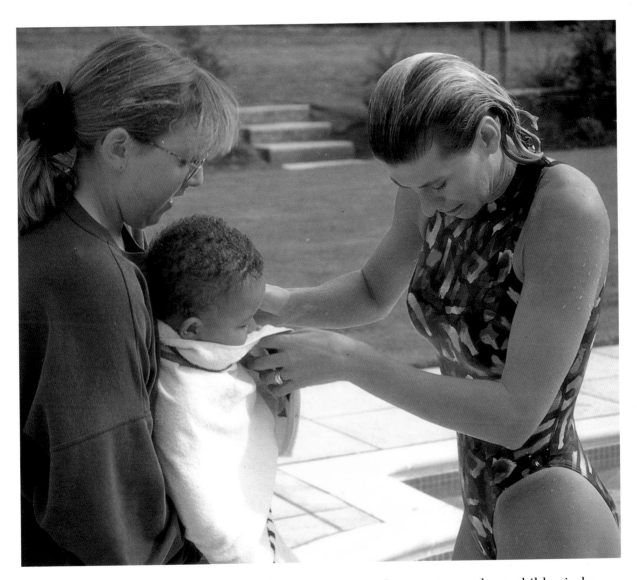

Elliott's nanny Sarah is just like part of the family.

One option that many mums choose is to employ a child-minder who looks after children in her own home. This allows a child to form a strong attachment with another regular face, and she will often get one-to-one attention. The number of children that a minder can look after is strictly regulated by the local council, and premises are also checked before approval is given and are likely to be spot checked at any time, so you can be as sure as is reasonably possible that your child will be safe. Although a child-minder will need a regular commitment to have your child for so many hours each week (and will expect to be paid a 'retainer' for the days you miss due to holidays or illness), they are often fairly flexible and able to mind at short notice should your circumstances demand it, and might even do evening babysitting.

Another alternative is to place your child in a nursery, where there will be more babies and children but also more helpers, more toys and more stimulation. Nursery care suits some children very well because they thrive in a busy environment and enjoy the company. Being with other children teaches them to share, as well as developing their social skills. Others, however, find it all a bit overpowering. Nursery care has improved over the years and many will now take babies from as young as three months by which time they will have had their first inoculations.

You might be able to afford a nanny either to live in or just to come to work each day. Different considerations apply here. Since the person will be in your home all day, you have to be sure that it is someone you are comfortable with. My own experience is that paper qualifications are not the be all and end all when it comes to finding the most suitable person to look after your child. Sarah, who looks after Elliott, is a family friend and not yet fully qualified, but we couldn't wish for a better nanny. Elliott adores her and she has fitted into our family very well.

Make sure that you interview all prospective nannies thoroughly and let your instincts guide you when it comes to making a decision. Always follow up references before you introduce a stranger into your household.

A similar but cheaper alternative is to employ an au pair. These are usually foreign girls who want to work here to learn to speak English, so you might have a language barrier to overcome, but they are very flexible and generally happy to fit in with whatever a family requests.

Whichever kind of child care you opt for there are certain questions you should ask.

- Is my potential child minder registered with the local authorities? (If the answer to this is no, look elsewhere.)
- Do I feel comfortable with this person?
- Does my child like her?
- Can I afford it?
- Is it close enough to my workplace to ensure that I can drop off my

baby in time to get to work without having to get up at the crack of dawn, and can collect him quickly if he is ill during the day?

- Do the other children in her care seem happy?
- Is the place clean, and safe? For instance, are there locks on cupboard doors, is there a safety gate over the stairs, and at the kitchen door, is there a fire guard? In Scotland the law states that anyone looking after a young child must have a fire guard fitted, while in England there is a Duty of Care which means that if a child falls on an unprotected fire – including that in her own home – she can sue the owners, and that could mean her own parents.

If you can choose a minder or nursery that has been recommended to you by a satisfied mum that, of course, is the ideal. Word of mouth is by far the best recommendation. But if this is your first foray into the world of parenting and you don't know where to start ask your Social Services office for a list of places with vacancies or talk to your health visitor.

If you have older children

You will need to make plans about where your older child or children will stay while you are in hospital. Even if you are intending to be in and out within a day, you will still need to arrange for someone to take care of them for that time, and to make provision for an overnight stay, just in case.

Obviously you should not leave your children with someone they do not know very well, and if they haven't stayed away from home overnight on their own before it might be a good idea to have a 'dry run' just in case. Try not to build it up into a big drama, but instil a pleasant sense of anticipation, and make it a treat so that they don't feel that they are being pushed out of the way.

The home front

No matter how fit and well you feel after you have had your baby, there are going to be times when the domestic routine starts to slip. A bit of judicious ground work now can save a crisis later, and more importantly it will mean that you and your partner will be able to give your full attention to your new baby.

Fill the freezer with bread, some complete meals such as pies and casseroles that need the minimum of attention to finish off, and some emergency rations such as fish portions, chops and pizzas. Don't forget vegetables. Freeze a couple of gourmet dishes, too, so that if you have a particularly fraught day you can sit down to a delicious meal in the evening. Stock up your storecupboard with tins of tuna, tomatoes, sweetcorn, whatever is your taste, plus lots of rice and pasta for quick meals, and basics such as tea, coffee, sugar, flour. Don't forget the essentials of toilet roll, soap, washing powder, washing up liquid, kitchen towels, plastic bags . . . But if all this planning sounds just a little too 'mumsy' for your style, don't forget that take-aways are an excellent stand-by in an emergency and there is no need to feel guilty if you send out for food once in a while.

Some women find that as their due date approaches they get the urge to springclean the house – part of the nesting instinct I suppose. If you feel like this, don't overdo it. Don't climb up a ladder to clean the bedrooms windows, and remember that bending is not as easy as it used to be. Get someone else to move the heavy furniture out of the way, and to carry the vacuum cleaner upstairs for you. Having said that, if you are the sort of person who bothers about dust, you will rest easier if you know that you have left a clean house behind you. Do what cleaning and tidying you can, and brief your partner on what needs to be done while you are away.

Phone numbers you might want to keep handy
Even the calmest of people can panic when confronted with an imminent birth, so plan ahead and pin a list of essential numbers by the phone.
GP.
Midwife.
Hospital labour ward.
Taxi firm.
Your partner's workplace.
Whoever is going to look after your older children.
Your parents.
Your partner's parents.
Anyone else who will want to know what you have had, when and how heavy.

Business matters

I knew I was expecting a boy, so I was able to buy the birth announcement cards in advance and write the addresses on the envelopes. Then all I had to do was to fill in the details once Elliott was born. I am not at all superstitious and had no qualms about doing this. If, however, you think (like Julia) that it is tempting fate, you can at least write a list of names and phone numbers of people to be called with the good news, so that your partner does not have to start rummaging through address books.

Make sure that you have claimed all you can from the DSS and that any details that need finalising with your employer are well in hand. Details of benefits are in Chapter 2.

Setting up a nursery

One of the most exciting jobs is getting a room ready for your new arrival. The shops are full of beautiful equipment and furnishings specially designed for babies, and it would be easy to spend a fortune getting everything just right.

There is no need to spend a lot of money on your baby's room – unless you want to, of course. He or she will enjoy colour and variety, but will appreciate £2 a roll end-of-line paper just as much as the designer-label £10 a roll equivalent. Similarly while it is nice for you for the room to have matching paper, curtains and bedding, the baby won't care as long as he is comfortable. What is important is that you choose decor that will provide lots for your baby to look at when he is awake, but that can also provide a calm, restful place to sleep. A child's bedroom should be a happy place that he enjoys, not somewhere he is sent as a punishment. If your budget won't stretch very far, plain painted walls are easy to keep clean and finished off with a

Elliott's bedroom.

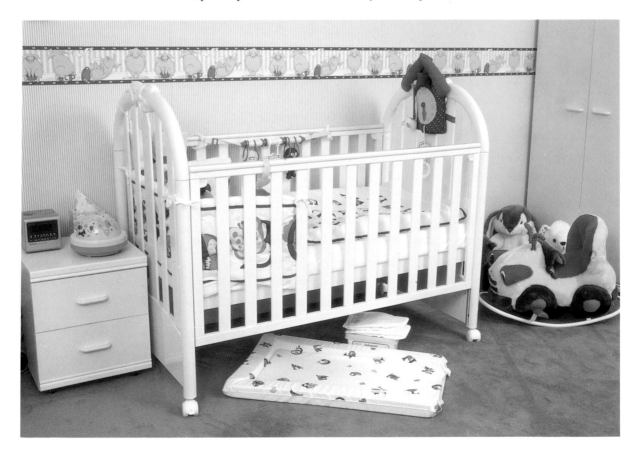

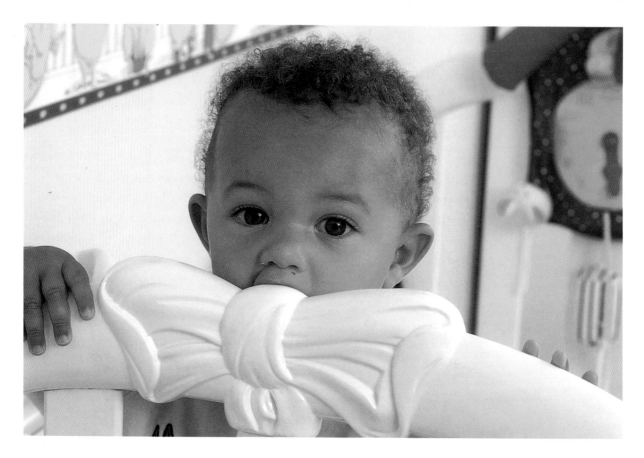

colourful border print they can look lovely – but you should be warned that many a baby thinks that it is a great game to pick off a border that you have thoughtfully placed at his height! You can also buy transfers and sticky scenes which are a simple and relatively cheap way of brightening up an otherwise plain room.

This is why you need to ensure that you use non-toxic paint on a cot!

Choose bright colours and don't feel that a boy has to have a blue room and a girl has to have pink. Be bold! Make sure that any paint you use is non-toxic.

Decorating a nursery is great fun, but don't go mad. Don't over-stretch yourself, or stand on a box to hang the curtains. You will probably find that rubbing down the paint on the skirting board is beyond you, too, so get some help, and don't let yourself become over-tired.

Buying equipment

A checklist of equipment you will need can be found at the end of the book, but here are some pointers you might like to bear in mind.

Carrycot.

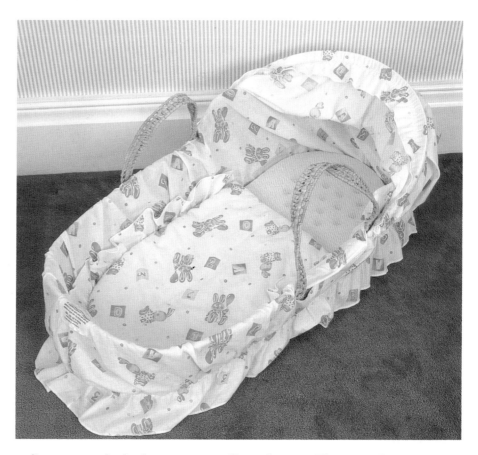

Starting with the basics, you will need a cot. There is a huge range available and they vary tremendously in style and cost, so choose whatever suits your taste and pocket. Buy one that has a drop side that runs smoothly and quietly. Most will have an adjustable base that can be lowered as your baby learns to stand, but which still leaves room underneath for some storage. You will need a mattress and again these vary quite a lot. Buy one that has a waterproof cover and breathing holes at the head end. Even if you buy a second-hand cot you should ideally get a new mattress. You won't need a pillow until your baby is at least one year old, and be wary of cot bumpers.

Some people like to have a Moses basket or baby nest so that they move the baby from room to room with them during the day. Alternatively a carrycot can be used for this, although if you get it wet while you are out this might be a problem. Special cot sheets are available and those with fitted corners are particularly useful, but cut-down or folded standard single bed sheets will do just as well. Several thinner layers are better than one thick one, so that you can adjust the bedding to suit the climate. Baby nests, duvets and quilts should be avoided for very young babies. They are often too warm and so cause over-heating, and might cause a child to suffocate. Your baby's bedroom should be well-ventilated but not draughty. A comfortable 19°C (65°F) is ideal. I bought a small portable radiator for Elliott's room which is thermostatically controlled and comes on when our central heating goes off, and ensures that his room is a constant temperature. I also bought a room thermometer via my health visitor, which she was able to sell me at a discount price, and which enabled me to make sure that Elliott's room was never too hot or too cold.

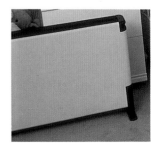

Thermostatically controlled radiator.

Next, somewhere to change nappies. Special changing units are available which incorporate a table top, cupboard for storage and fold-out flaps for baby lotion, wipes and so on. If you prefer, you can place a changing mat on top of a table or chest of drawers at first, but beware that even tiny babies can roll at an alarming rate, so use a mat which has raised sides. Better still, use the floor.

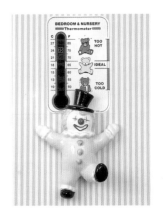

Room thermometer.

You will need somewhere to store your baby's clothes. At this stage a chest of drawers will do, as few if any baby clothes need hanging up. A small bookcase is useful not just for books and ornaments but also for things that you need readily to hand, such as baby wipes, cotton wool, or a favourite cuddly toy. Be sure that potentially dangerous things are moved upwards as your baby starts to crawl and stand.

You might like to consider thick curtains and a night light or dimmer switch. However, if a baby is tired he will sleep wherever he is and whatever the lighting. (Conversely, of course, if he is *not* tired there is nothing you can do to make him drop off . . .) Similarly, there is really no need to tiptoe around the house when your baby is asleep. The quieter you are the quieter you have to be, but remember that when your baby was in hospital he had to sleep through the noise of trolleys rattling up and down the corridor at all hours, other babies crying, visitors chatting, nurses talking to other 'inmates', so don't think you have to put your own life on hold just because Junior has gone to bed. Elliott has a radio on in his bedroom just very quietly in the background, which he seems to enjoy.

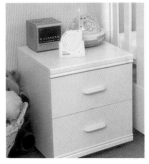

A simple chest of drawers is all you need to store your baby's clothes at first. Elliott's is also used as a place to keep his radio, night light and listening device.

Cot activity centres are useful as your baby grows older and can press the buttons and make things happen. You might be *really* lucky

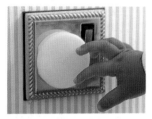

This socket cover keeps little fingers at bay, while also acting as a gentle night light.

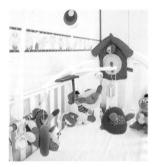

Make sure that your baby has plenty to look at in his room.

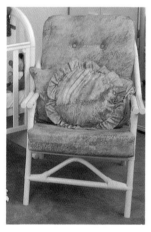

A comfortable chair is a useful addition to a well-equipped nursery.

and have the sort of baby who will wake and amuse himself with it until it is time to get up! Mobiles, too, will catch your baby's eye from a very early age and give endless pleasure.

It is also useful to have a chair in your baby's room so that you have somewhere to sit for those night feeds and to cuddle and settle your baby at other times.

Next transport. You must have your baby (and indeed older children) restrained in the car at all times. The safest place for a new baby to travel is in the back of the car in a rearward-facing car seat, one attached by special fixings or held by an inertia-reel seatbelt. There are some very lightweight first stage car seats available which you can pick up with one hand even with the baby in it, and these are wonderful because they mean that you do not have to disturb a sleeping child at the end of your journey and you can carry him into friends' homes, shops, restaurants or wherever else you need to go. One step up from these are seats which can be used facing either forwards or backwards and will last the child several years until he reaches the maximum weight recommended by the manufacturer. There are also seats which are designed only to be used facing forwards, but which are bigger and so last a little longer before you have to invest in booster seats.

If you have a carrycot that you wish to put in the car you should install special restraining straps, and also put the cover on for the journey. If you have to travel in someone else's car wedge the carrycot on the floor between the front and back seats.

Whether you buy a pushchair, pram or something that will convert from one to the other depends on your lifestyle. If you have a car make sure that what you buy will fit in the boot. If you do a lot of walking it pays to invest in a sturdier pram that will accommodate shopping and provide a comfortable ride. Broadly speaking, the choices are these.

A traditional pram is by far the warmest option, it is sturdy and will last a baby longer because it is usually bigger than some of the combination alternatives. However, the drawbacks are that it does take up quite a bit of space and cannot be used once the baby is much beyond one year old.

A three-in-one combination pram/pushchair is useful because it is possible to buy something that will last your baby from his first outing until he gives up riding altogether. This type tends to come with a detachable carrycot section which as I have already said makes a useful bed for the first few weeks of a baby's life as it is easily portable. It also has the advantage that you can put the wheels back on it to rock the baby to sleep if needs be. As the baby grows you can convert the pram into a rearward-facing pushchair which can be reclined until your baby can sit up unsupported and without slumping. Finally it can be turned around to make a front-facing pushchair.

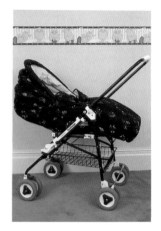

There are other models of pushchair which can face forwards and backwards, or just forwards, and there are also strollers, lightweight pushchairs that can be easily folded with one hand and are excellent if you travel by bus a lot. You can even get a car seat which can be clipped on to a frame to become a pushchair. Whatever style of pushchair you eventually decide on, you will also need a waterproof cover and a sunshade.

A pram that converts into a pushchair is an excellent investment.

Many items can be picked up relatively cheaply second-hand and because babies grow so quickly much will be in good condition. Don't, however, buy a second-hand car seat unless you are absolutely certain that it has not been involved in any accident. Even if it shows no sign of damage it might have become weakened by a crash, and this is one area where it definitely does not pay to cut corners. Whatever equipment you buy, make sure it has the British Standard kite mark on it. Be particularly careful if you are buying second hand.

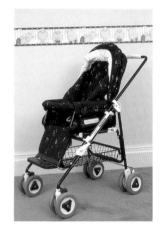

If you are working to a tight budget, when you are investing in furniture such as chests of drawers, cupboards and wardrobes, try to buy that which will grow with the child rather than things which are obviously tailor-made for babies. All equipment should be easy to clean. Don't forget it is possible to hire equipment if you don't think you will need it for very long.

A baby box to keep all your equipment together in one handy place is useful. This doesn't have to be a specially made, expensive affair. A plastic toolbox from any DIY chain store is just as good, or even a large ice-cream tub, perhaps covered with the nursery wallpaper to disguise its humble origins.

It is a good idea just to buy the essentials at first. You are bound to be given presents, and until you have had your baby at home for a while you won't really have a clear idea of what you need. Consult the checklists at the end of the book and talk to mums who are old hands to find out what you really need and what are just nice extras that you could manage without.

Don't forget that unless you have a huge house the presence of your baby will be felt in every room. Toys will need to be kept in your living room and sticky fingers will reach into every crevice. As well as making sure that your living space is safe by fitting cupboard locks, protectors on sharp corners, socket covers and so on, your furnishings will need a bit of attention. If you have a light coloured suite you might want to cover it with a colourful throw to protect it. If you happen to be decorating, choose 'childproof' colours and designs that will not show every mark, and make sure that carpets and other fabrics can be cleaned.

One final thought: you might prefer to keep your baby in your own bedroom at first. This is very handy for night-time feeds, and it is reassuring to know you are close at hand. Be careful though not to forget that it is your partner's room too, and he might resent the intrusion if it goes on for too long. Elliott has been in his own room since he was about two weeks old, but for reassurance I had a baby listener that was so sensitive I could even hear him breathing if I wanted to.

Chapter 7

PREPARING FOR THE BIRTH

I am not going to tell you too much about what happens to your body during pregnancy, or go into details about the 'mechanics' of giving birth. There are plenty of other books around that do that. But I want to take a look at what you need to know in order to have an informed pregnancy, and to make the right decision about the sort of labour and birth you would ideally like to have.

Tests – and results

From the first time you visit your GP to have your pregnancy confirmed you will undergo various tests and procedures along the way to ensure that you and your baby are well. If you are a healthy person who seldom visits a doctor it can be rather disconcerting suddenly to find yourself the subject of all this attention, so if you know in advance what it is all about you will not be worried by it. However, all these tests are routine, and you should not be concerned if they are offered to you. Precise details of antenatal care and the testing offered and available varies throughout the country so check with your own practice what their policy is. The following gives you some guidance, however.

BLOOD TESTS

At your first antenatal consultation you will have a blood test which will be used:

a. to establish your blood group, that is to determine to which ABO group you belong and whether your blood is Rhesus-positive or negative;

b. to check your haemoglobin level to ensure that you are not anaemic. If you are, you will be prescribed a course of iron tablets to help this. Your haemoglobin level will be tested again at intervals during your pregnancy;

c. to look for other evidence of infection, Hepatitis B and syphilis as standard (and random HIV tests are carried out on pregnant women and babies, purely to gather statistics);

d. to test for immunity to rubella (German measles).

Between the 15th and 18th weeks of your pregnancy you will be offered a blood test which checks for levels of a protein called alphafetoprotein in your blood. This protein is produced by the baby and a small amount is present in your blood. If the level detected is not as anticipated:

a. double the amount might indicate twins;

b. a higher than expected level might be an indication of spina bifida;

c. a lower than expected level might indicate that the baby has Down's syndrome.

There is also another blood test known as the Triple Test which identifies double the amount of Down's babies to the previous tests, and is based on the presence of hormones called human gonadotrophin and oestriol and analysis of results is based on the mother's age. This test must be carried out at 16 weeks. A positive result means that there is higher than average risk that the baby has Down's syndrome, but does *not* mean that it definitely has.

AMNIOCENTESIS

Amniocentesis is offered to all women who are at risk of having a baby with some defect, for instance if something is indicated by a blood test, if there have been problems with an earlier pregnancy or if her age suggests that she is more likely to have problems. The test is carried out by having a thin needle inserted into your abdomen and a sample of amniotic fluid taken. This is uncomfortable but it does not hurt, although you will feel sore for a day or so afterwards and will have to take things easy for a while. This test can be used to detect spina bifida, Down's syndrome and other genetic disorders, as well as determining the sex of the baby. There is a miscarriage rate of about 1 per cent.

CVS

Chorionic Villus Sampling can also be used for detecting Down's syndrome. It involves taking a sample of tissue from that surrounding the unborn baby and can be done between eight and ten weeks. However, it has a lower accuracy rate than amniocentesis and a carries higher risk of miscarriage.

ULTRASOUND SCAN

An ultrasound scan creates an image of your insides by using sound echoes reflected back from your internal organs. It is used to check that all is well with your baby. A scan is not usually offered until the 16th week, although some health authorities offer an earlier scan to confirm the expected date of delivery. Even at a very few weeks the baby's heartbeat can be detected. An ultrasound scan is completely painless. All that happens is that a hand-held device similar to a microphone is rubbed over your bump.

It is a lovely feeling being able to see your baby before it is born. At first the image on the screen may look just like a variety of shades of grey, but the radiographer who does the test will be able to point out your baby's limbs, face, spine, heart – even the four separate chambers of the heart – and will be able to take accurate measurements to confirm that your dates are correct and that the baby is growing at the expected rate, as well as providing information on the position and size of the placenta. Depending on how the baby is lying it is also possible to determine its sex although you may not automatically be told this, even if you want to know. Again policy varies between hospitals.

The early scan I had of Elliott suggested that he had a small kidney problem, and that my placenta was lying low which might have meant my having a Caesarian. As a precaution I was given a scan every month but thankfully my placenta moved to its rightful place before the end of my pregnancy and Elliott is perfectly well. It was reassuring to know that my condition could be monitored so closely.

Your medical notes

Because you will see several different medics during pregnancy – GP, midwife, health visitor, hospital staff – you will be given one set of notes to carry around with you which will be updated by each person who sees you. This ensures consistency of care without duplication. However, just because you get to keep your notes during your

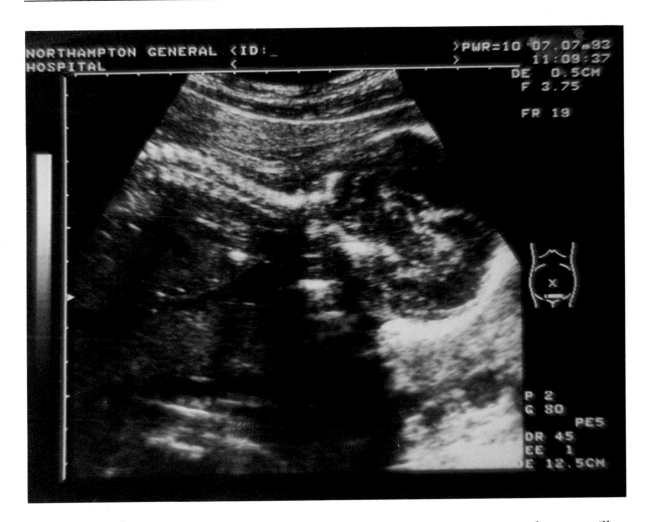

Elliott's spine can be seen in the top left-hand corner of this scan picture.

Photograph: Sharron Davies collection.

pregnancy doesn't mean that they are written in a way that you will automatically understand. They are a ready record of your history, your present condition and your future requirements and expectations (in every sense).

Your notes will record your personal details, name, address, phone number, age, date of birth, occupation, marital status, religion, next of kin, GP, midwife, consultant, details of your family's medical history if relevant (if you are a twin, for instance), and your own past medical and surgical history, including any operations or blood transfusions you have had, details of your periods and previous contraception used, if you are taking any medication, if you have any allergies and whether or not you smoke and drink. Your height, weight and, curiously, shoe size might be recorded too.

If you have had any previous pregnancies these will also be noted, along with details of the outcome – if the pregnancy went to full term, where your baby was born, after how many weeks, if you had any problems either during pregnancy or delivery, weight and sex of any babies and whether or not you breastfed.

All blood tests and their results will be recorded, plus any other tests you undergo such as amniocentesis. Your midwife or GP should tell you what is being recorded on your notes, and if you see anything you don't understand you should ask. The following highlights some of the abbreviations and medical jargon you might see in your notes:

LMP	*Last monthly period.*
EDD	*Expected date of delivery.*
BP	*Blood pressure.*
Hb	*Haemoglobin.*
NAD	*Nothing abnormal detected.*
+ or tr	*Trace of either sugar or protein detected in a urine sample.*
Height/fundus	*Measurement of how far the top of your uterus is above your pubic bone.*
PP	*Presenting part of the baby, ie the part that is coming first. Head down is usually noted as c or ceph for cephalic or Vx for vertex. Bottom first is noted as Br for breech.*
Position	*How the crown of the baby's head (O for occiput) is lying in relation to your body: pointing left or right (L or R), to the front (A for anterior), sideways (T, transverse or L, lateral) or backwards (P, posterior).*
Engagement	*Indication of whether or not the baby has moved down into the pelvis. E is engaged, NE is not engaged.*
FH	*Fetal heart; FHH – fetal heart heard, FHNH – fetal heart not heard.*
FMF	*Fetal movements felt.*
Oedema	*Swelling.*

Writing a birth plan

Every pregnancy is different. Even if you are preparing for the birth of your second or third child, there is no guarantee that this pregnancy will be the same as the first, or that your delivery will be the same. If you are a first-timer no one can *really* tell you what labour is like or what it feels like to give birth, so the best you can do is to gather information together from books, literature provided by your GP and midwife, and feedback from friends who have been through it, then make up your own mind. It is a good idea to make a birth plan, because when the time comes you won't want to have to make any decisions about the attention you are receiving; you will need all your energies – mental and physical – to concentrate on the matter in hand.

Whatever you decide, you must keep an open mind and be prepared to be flexible. If you set your heart on a completely natural birth and have to have a Caesarean section you could be deeply disappointed and have your confidence shaken, so think about what you would like to happen in an ideal situation but be aware that when the time comes your best route is just to 'go with the flow'. Be prepared to change your plan as your labour progresses. It is important that your partner knows what your wishes are so that if you find you are not able to speak for yourself for whatever reason you can be sure that nothing will be done to you that you would not want. It is worth bearing in mind that some of your requests might meet with opposition either because they are unusual and do not fit in with what the hospital considers to be the norm, or because medical opinion advises against them. Be reasonable. Trust the professionals and make informed decisions.

Consider the following:

1. Where do you want to have your baby? The assumption tends to be that every woman will want to have her baby in a hospital, but that is not always true. If you want to have your baby at home you might have to try very hard to persuade the authorities to agree. However, stick to your guns because you are legally entitled to have your baby where you want it. Even so there may be very sound medical reasons for advising you to opt for a hospital birth. For instance, if you have been unwell during pregnancy or if you had complications with a previous delivery. Alternatively, you

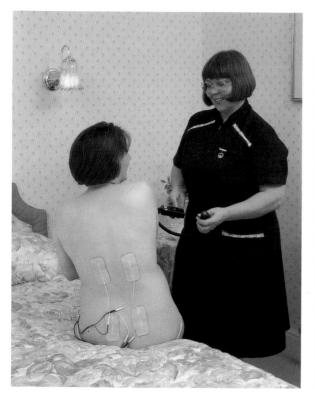

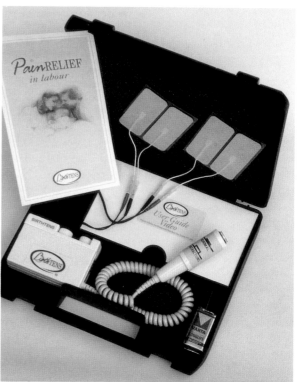

might want to go to a hospital that is outside your health authority, for example to a hospital that has a pool for water births. Again, there should be no problem with this because you are within your rights to insist.

2. Who do you want to be with you? The most obvious choice is the baby's father, but this is not always the case. If you want someone else there as well or instead of him, check what the hospital's policy is. You can, of course, opt to give birth with just the medical staff present. You might also like to check with the hospital who will be present from their side and whether students are likely to be there. If you object to what they suggest you should say so.

3. Are you able to take in any personal equipment such as triangular wedges, cushions, beanbags, birthing stool, TENS machine, or are they available? I took in a tape recorder so that Elliott could be born to music – and Derek was most insistent that I held on until he had found precisely the right track!

A TENS machine increases your body's pain-relieving substances called endorphines, and blocks the pain pathways to your brain, therefore reducing the intensity of the anticipated pain. The upper pads are placed just below your bra strap and the lower ones on the sacral dimples.

Photograph: Bounty Pain Management.

4. What sort of pain relief do you want? Check with the hospital what is available, because not all will offer the same. If you want an epidural you should say so as soon as possible, because it needs an anaesthetist to be present for it to be administered and there may not be one available if you leave it to the last minute.

5. How do you feel about other intervention – monitoring of the baby during labour, forceps, Caesarian section, enemas, induction and acceleration, episiotomy and stitches, use of Syntometrine to speed up the delivery of the placenta? I had been very sure that I did not want an episiotomy unless it was absolutely vital so I tore slightly. I had my stitches taken out as early as was safely possible because they were at the front and annoyed me when I moved.

6. Do you want to be able to walk around during labour? This will have some bearing on the type of pain relief you choose.

7. In what position do you want to give birth?

8. Where do you want the baby put immediately after delivery – on to your stomach? Do you want to feed him straight away?

9. How long do you want to stay in hospital?

My experiences

I had my maternity care under the Domino system, which allowed me to have the same midwife looking after me all the way through. In the end she was with me at home for about 14 hours and came to the hospital with me to deliver Elliott. Because of who I am, many people assumed that I would opt for a water birth. However, the NHS hospital where Elliott was born did not have the facilities, and although I could have hired a pool I decided against it and instead used my bath at home to provide pain relief as a compromise. Maybe next time . . .

While I was pregnant there was a lot of scaremongering in the press about the risks involved with a water birth because a baby delivered that way had subsequently died, albeit of causes not directly related to the use of a pool. I would not be put off by this because any competent midwife will take you out of the water if there is the slightest risk either to you or your baby.

At 11 pm one evening Derek rang my midwife to tell her that I had

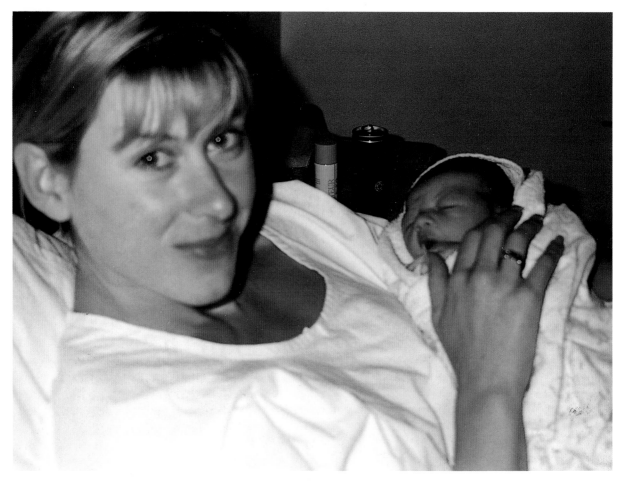

Proud mum with Elliott, less than an hour old.

Photograph: Sharron Davies collection.

gone into labour. She came over at about 3 am and stayed for three hours before going home to freshen up a little. I was having fairly regular contractions but was able to cope. She returned to take me into hospital at noon. By this time I was only half-way dilated because of my strong stomach muscles, a legacy of all the hard training I do, so I was advised to have an epidural. This gave me a rest, but I was aware of losing control of the situation. An epidural is usually topped up after a while but I asked for this not to be done so that by the time Elliott was finally born I had recovered about 50 per cent of sensation and I could feel what was happening. Elliott had the cord around his neck, but this was corrected between pushes. Here my strong muscles came into their own because I only had to push twice and suddenly Elliott was there. (Derek said afterwards that he was half expecting to need his baseball glove to catch him as he came out!)

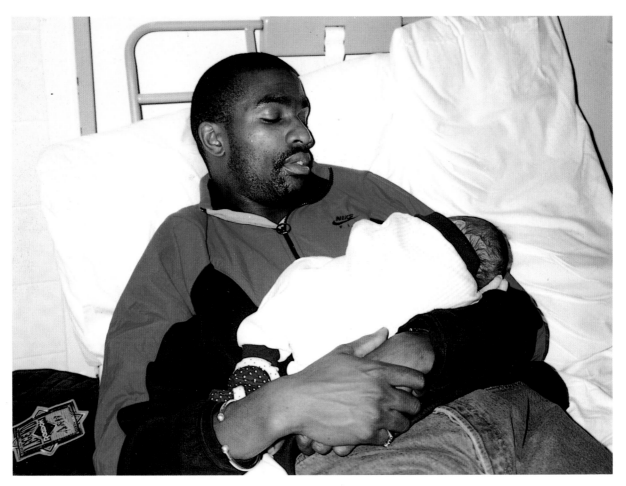

Proud dad – almost as tired as mum!

Photograph: Sharron Davies collection.

Elliott was delivered at 5.20 pm on 4 November, weighing in at a healthy 8 lb 4 oz, and handed to Derek while I was stitched (happily just a few), then I fed him about an hour later.

My biggest fear beforehand had been that I would do something to embarrass myself, but when the time came I couldn't have cared less. The support that Derek gave me was invaluable. He was with me the whole time and I wouldn't have liked to have gone through it without him. I also believe that I benefited from having the same midwife throughout, because I know that some women who have a long labour can go through several shifts and see many different faces. Midwives are very special people and doctors will often consult with them before making some decisions. You can put your trust in them. They have the experience of delivering babies every day of the week and are true professionals.

Chapter 8

POST-NATAL REGIME

The first few days when you arrive home with your new baby are very strange. You went into hospital as one half of a couple but you came out as part of a family, and that can take some getting used to. You will have to do some adapting and spend some time getting to know the new addition to the household, but you will be able to cope more easily if you are physically up to speed. Try to have an afternoon nap if at all possible. I know all the books say this, and all new mums laugh at the idea of having time to put their feet up for an hour, but believe me it is worth it. You feel so much better for taking a rest. I found that when Elliott took a nap I saw it as an opportunity to catch up on a few jobs and would rush around like a headless chicken trying to get things done – so don't do as I did, do as I say!

Before you leave hospital

Whether you have your baby and come out of the hospital on the same day or whether you stay for a few days will depend on how your delivery went, how quickly you recover and on your own wishes. While you are in hospital the staff will keep an eye on you, checking your tummy to see if your uterus is going down as it should, monitoring your temperature, administering any drugs you may need and generally making sure that you are fit and well. They will keep asking you if you have been to the toilet until you say 'yes'. You may well be putting it off, especially if you have had stitches, because you think you are going to burst open. Someone will always be on hand to answer any queries you have and to ease any worries, so don't be afraid to ask if you are unsure about anything. The hospital staff understand how daunting it is suddenly to be responsible for a new life. You will probably be shown how to change nappies, 'top and tail' your baby (that is to wash him) and depending on staffing levels,

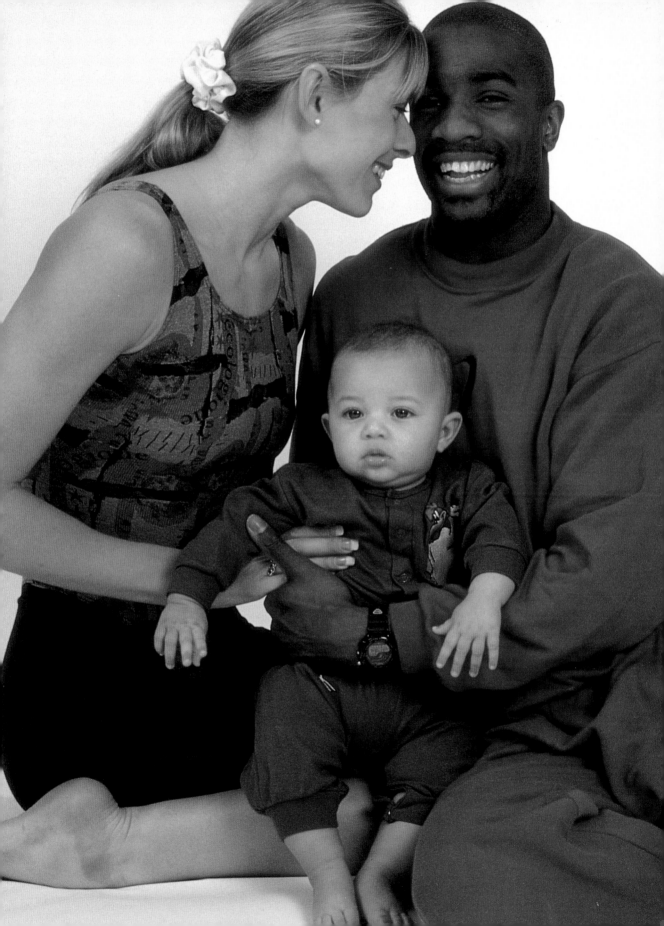

shown how to give him a bath and wash his hair (if he has any). Incidentally, a baby's fingernails seem to grow extremely quickly and if you are not vigilant he could scratch his face. A good tip is to trim them while he is asleep so that he can't struggle.

If you are breastfeeding your baby you will be given lots of advice and encouragement to do this properly and to find a position that suits you and your baby. I had always thought that breastfeeding was a perfectly natural thing and that babies instinctively knew what to do. It therefore came as something of a surprise to find out that a baby had to be 'taught'. If your baby doesn't 'latch on' properly it can be quite painful for you, as well as being frustrating for him if he is sucking away valiantly and not getting anywhere. Once you have learnt the technique, however, it is a rewarding experience, and you can be sure that you are giving your baby the best possible start in life. But, if you do not want to breastfeed for whatever reason, there is no need to feel guilty that you are failing in some way. It is your choice.

Another thing that surprises some new mums is that your full milk does not arrive as soon as your baby is born, which makes them anxious and upset because they feel that they are not producing enough to feed their baby. For the first three days you will only produce colostrum, a thick creamy liquid that is rich in nutrients and contains antibodies that will help your baby fight infection. Your full milk should 'come in' on the third day and from then on you should find you have a plentiful supply with which to feed. If you truly don't think you can keep up with the demands your baby is making on you, don't feel as if you have failed. Many women bring up happy and healthy babies without breastfeeding. While on this subject it is worth mentioning the benefits of expressing milk, either by hand or using a breast pump. This enables you to make up feeds that can then be given by someone else, which allows you to have a rest. Breast milk can also be frozen for use at a later date.

Take care of your nipples as they can get cracked and sore. Use breast pads to soak up any leaks and let the air get to your breasts as often as decency allows. It is a good idea to take some nipple cream into hospital with you.

Your baby will also be given a thorough check before you bring him home. A doctor will look at the colour of his skin to check for any blemishes or signs of jaundice, feel his tummy to check that his internal organs are in the right place and are the right size, and check that his cord is drying up nicely. She will listen to his heart and check his breathing, feel his pulse, look into his eyes and feel in his mouth, examine his genitals, check his spine and muscle tone and watch him kick his legs and arms. One of the checks that is slightly disturbing to you and your baby is the one to see that his hip joints work properly. This is done by holding his legs straight, then bending them at the knees and turning them out to the side to see if they lie completely flat. He will also be measured for length and head circumference, and will be weighed. Most babies lose weight immediately after they are born, but they should soon return to their birth weight.

Because Elliott is part Afro-Caribbean, he was tested for Sickle Cell disease, an inherited blood condition which affects some people of West African origin, and which results in chronic anaemia and periods of pain due to blockage of the blood vessels. It used to be the case that an injection of vitamin K was given to all newborn babies as a matter of course as a precaution against haemorrhage. However, recently there has been concern that there is a link between this and childhood cancer. An oral dose is thought to be less controversial than the intra-muscular dose, but that is not licensed in Britain. In some areas of the country vitamin K is still administered routinely, often with little or no explanation, so make sure you know what is being done to your baby and if you are in any doubt, ask.

Getting back into shape

It might sound a rather obvious thing to say, but having a baby is a very physical experience and you cannot expect your body to be exactly the same afterwards as it was before, but your new body is not necessarily worse just different. If you have stretch marks they will never disappear altogether but they will fade slightly in time. However, you can tone up flabby thighs and flatten your tummy with some exercises. You won't be able to get into your jeans for your journey home from hospital but with a little bit of effort it won't be long before you can. My vanity led me to squeeze into my jeans on the third day, stitches and all. I went shopping and found after a while that I could hardly walk for the pain! The important thing is to take it steadily. Your body is like a big elastic band. If you stretch it to the extreme it may not go back exactly as it was, but it will go 98 per cent of the way – and only you will notice the difference.

After the birth of your baby the hospital staff will give you advice on what exercises you should do, and you should follow their instructions. However, it is worth remembering that any exercise sheets you are given will be written to be safe for absolutely anyone, even those women who have never taken any exercise at all. You can of course do these routines, but if you have maintained a reasonable level of fitness throughout your pregnancy you will want and need to do something a little more testing.

At what stage you can take up any exercise will depend on the type of labour and delivery you had. If you had a 20-hour labour and a lot of stitches then obviously you will need to take it more gradually than if you were in and out in 5 hours. A good indication is that once your bleeding has stopped you can resume a reasonable routine. If your find your bleeding restarts or worsens you should ease off and check with your GP or midwife.

I was quite determined to get back to my pre-pregnancy level of fitness as quickly as possible, and was back on an exercise bike when Elliott was three days old. I was working out in the gym a bit too soon, however, and I got very upset and disillusioned when I couldn't make my body do what I wanted it to when using weights.

Even if you do no other exercises at all, don't forget to look after your pelvic floor. You will find details of this exercise in Chapter 4.

Post-natal exercises

I found that as soon as I started to exercise again after Elliott was born I felt an immediate benefit, not just physically but also mentally. The exercises illustrated here are the ones that I did and all recommendations given are based on my own experience. Obviously you should not do anything that you do not feel comfortable with and if you are in any doubt about whether or not you should do any of the exercises or stretches, check with your GP or midwife.

THIGH SQUEEZE

You will find that many of the exercises described in Chapter 4 are good for getting you back into shape. This one for your inner thigh, for instance, can be done during pregnancy and after with equal success.

Lie on one side with your knees bent and your feet together, and lean up on your lower arm. Slowly raise and lower your upper leg without twisting your hip. Feel the muscles in your inner thighs working. Repeat 10 times on each side.

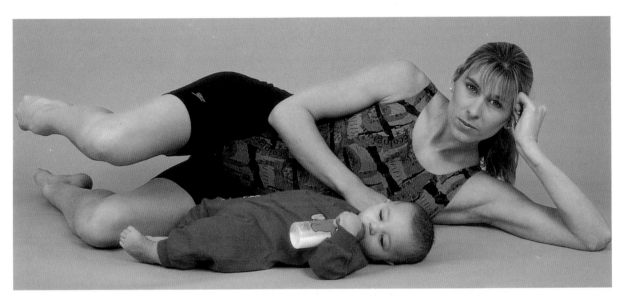

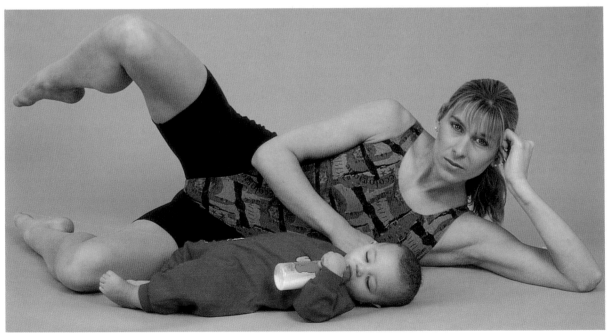

Even feeding time can be exercise time! Keep yourself fit and supple after your baby is born by keeping up your stretching exercises.

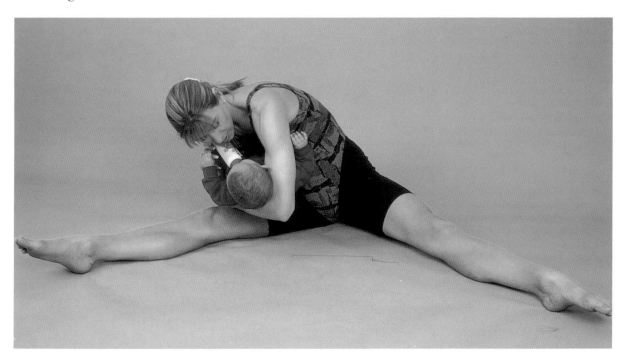

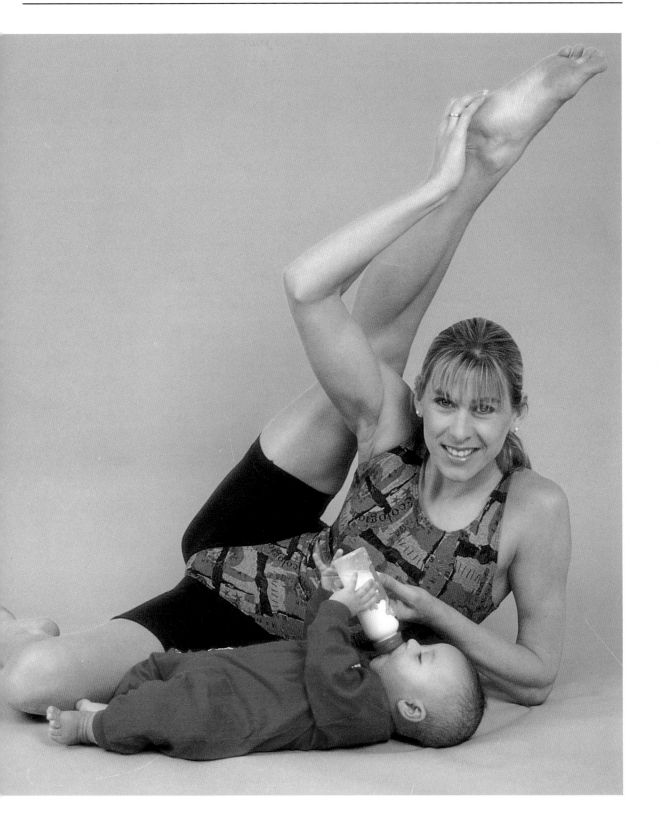

INNER SIDE LEG RAISE

This sounds more complicated that it actually is, so be guided by the pictures! You should feel a squeeze in your inner thighs. Flexing your foot makes it harder.

Lie on your left side with your legs straight then lean up supporting your weight on your left arm. Bend your right knee and put your right foot on the floor in front of you. Lift and raise your left leg slowly, keeping it straight. Repeat 10 to 20 times on both sides.

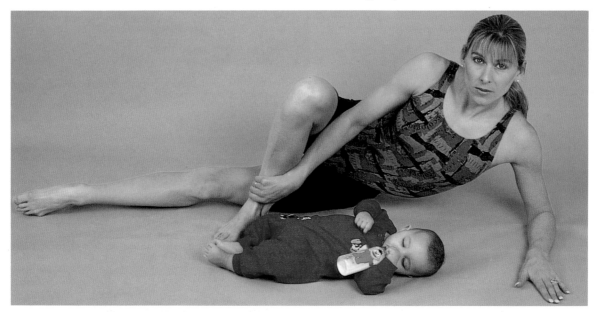

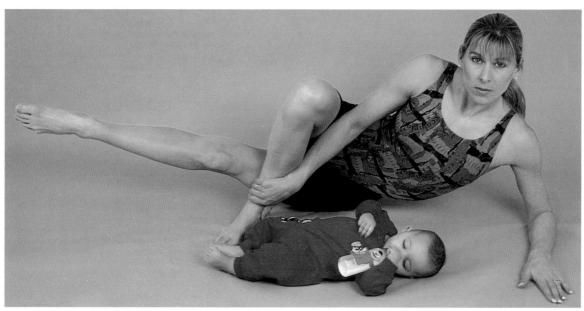

REVERSE PRESS-UP

Your baby will find it highly amusing to watch you exercising - so why not let him join in? Use him here as an appealing weight!

Lie on your back with your knees bent. Hold your baby securely in both hands and gradually raise and lower him as you straighten and bend your arms. Repeat eight to 10 times.

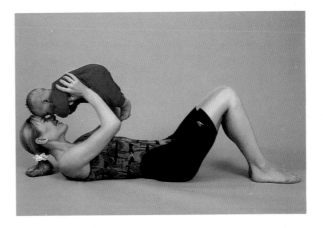

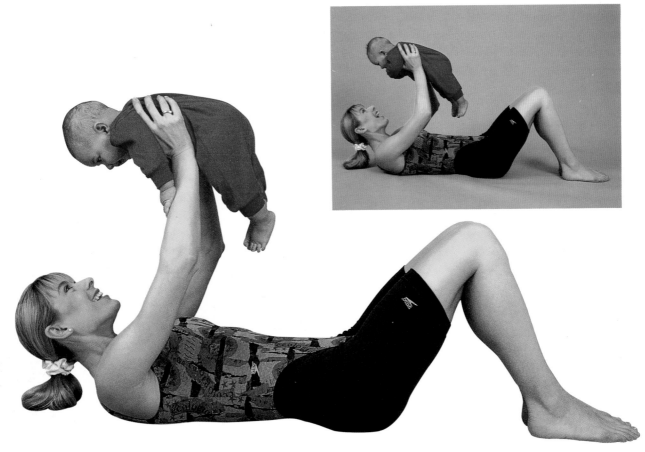

SIT-UPS

When you do sit-ups you should always bend
your knees to avoid straining your back.
There is no need to do this exercise at great
speed. To make this exercise easier, anchor
your feet under the sofa or get someone to
hold them.

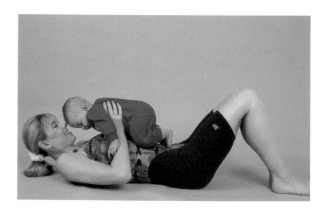

*If you are not going
to hold your baby as
you do this exercise,
put your hands on
your temples and
keep your elbows*
*back, or cross your
hands on your chest.
Use your stomach
muscles to pull you
into a sitting position
then gently unroll*

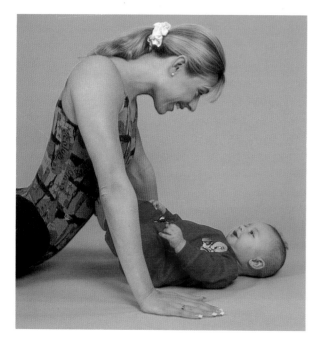

BACK ARCH

You met this exercise in Chapter 4, but now
that you no longer have your bump to
consider you should find it much easier. It is
an excellent complement to the sit-ups as it
stretches the abdominal muscles you have just
worked.

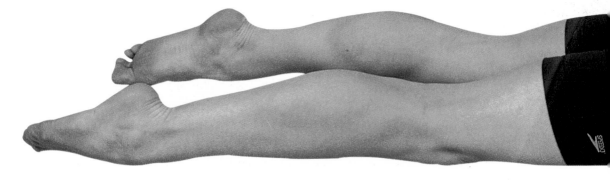

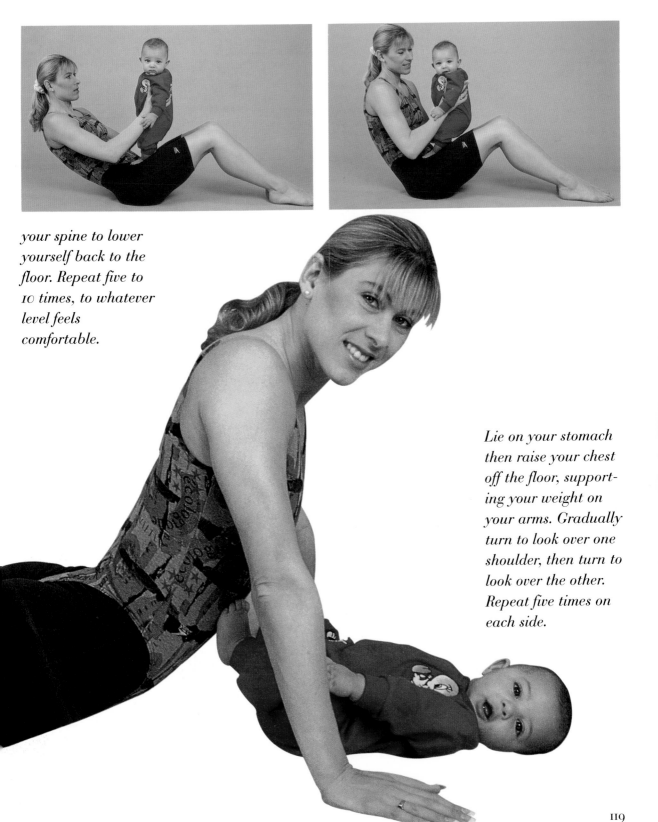

your spine to lower
yourself back to the
floor. Repeat five to
10 times, to whatever
level feels
comfortable.

Lie on your stomach
then raise your chest
off the floor, support-
ing your weight on
your arms. Gradually
turn to look over one
shoulder, then turn to
look over the other.
Repeat five times on
each side.

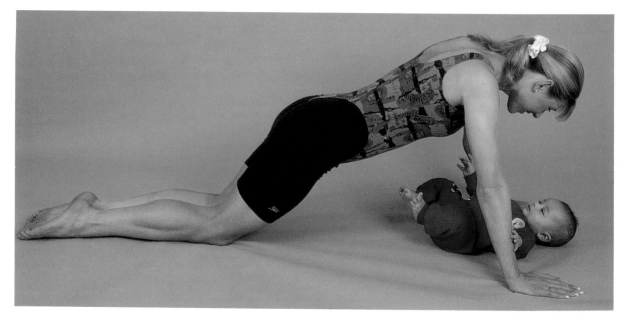

SUPPORTED PRESS-UP
Bend down and give your little one a kiss while working on the tone of your arms and shoulders.

Kneel on all fours but with your legs sloping rather than bent at 90°. Bend and straighten your arms in the manner of a press-up 15-20 times.

As you get stronger move your legs further back. The further they go, the harder the exercise. Repeat 10-20 times.

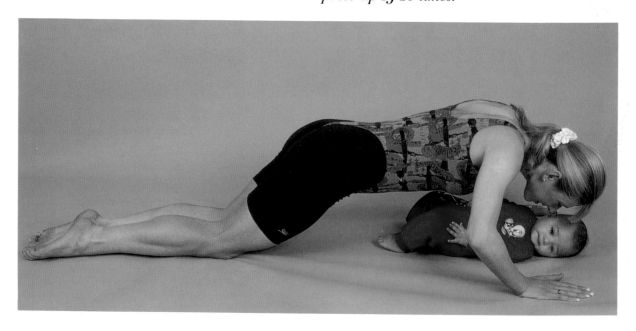

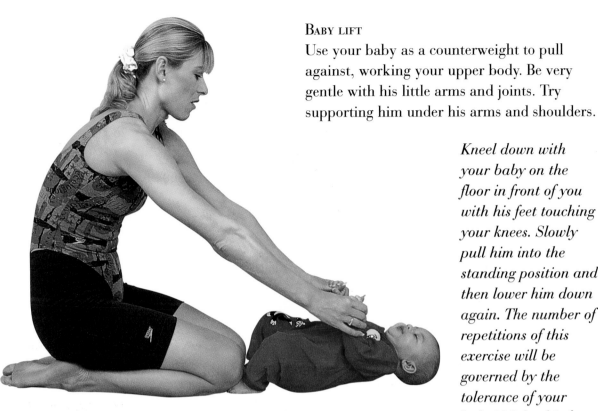

BABY LIFT

Use your baby as a counterweight to pull against, working your upper body. Be very gentle with his little arms and joints. Try supporting him under his arms and shoulders.

Kneel down with your baby on the floor in front of you with his feet touching your knees. Slowly pull him into the standing position and then lower him down again. The number of repetitions of this exercise will be governed by the tolerance of your baby! Make this fun. It is more of a game than serious exercise.

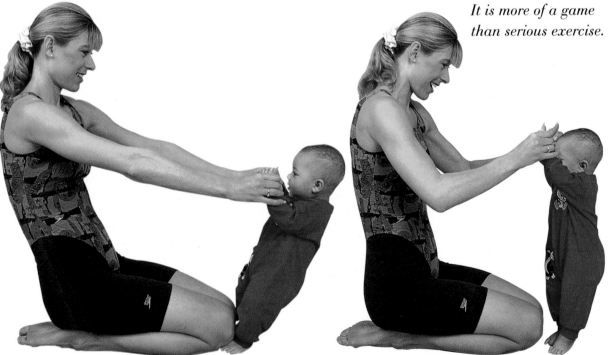

MINI LEG RAISES

This one can also be great fun for both of you, as well as being good for your thighs and bottom.

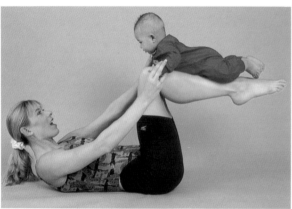

Lie on your back with your legs pulled in so your shins are parallel with the floor. Position your baby comfortably on your legs, straighten them slightly then bend again. Again, repeat until the novelty wears off.

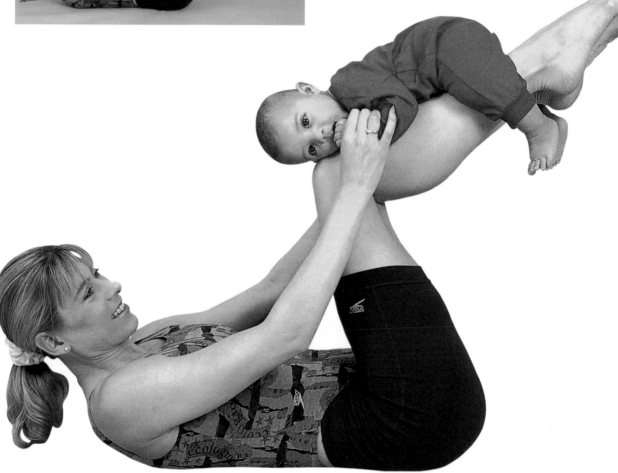

Water exercises

Swimming is one of the best forms of exercise you can get because it gives your whole body a thorough work-out while the water takes the strain for you. As well as ordinary swimming you might like to try the following exercises.

SWEEPS

This exercise is outlined in Chapter 4, but when you are pregnant you have to do it holding on to the side. Here it is shown free-standing which requires more balance.

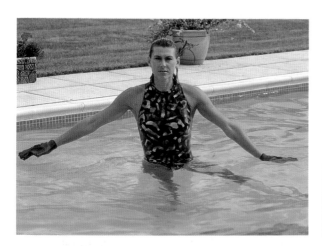

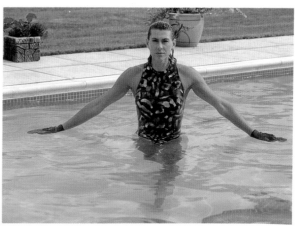

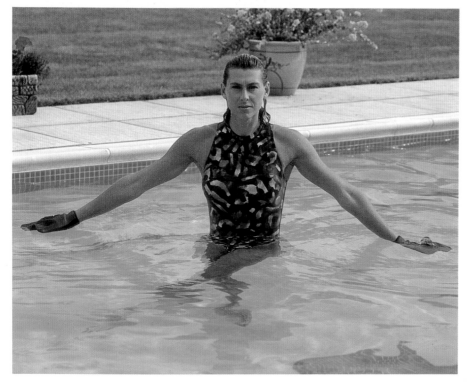

Stand in at least waist-high water with your arms out to your sides to help you balance. Sweep one leg across the other and back again. Repeat five to 10 times with each leg.

KNEE RAISES

This is another exercise that you can also do while you are pregnant, as long as you use the side of the pool for support. It works your hip flexors.

Standing in about waist-high water, raise and lower your knee five to 10 times with each leg.

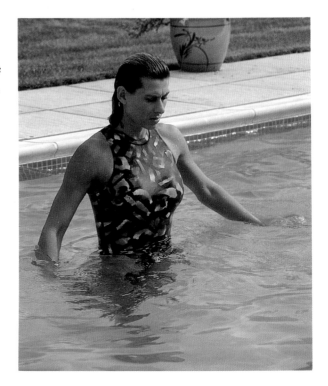

AIDED PRESS-UP

This is a good post-natal exercise but you could also do it in the early stages of your pregnancy before you bump starts to get in the way.

Place your hands flat on the floor outside the pool, then using the muscles of your arms and shoulders pull yourself out of the water until your arms are straight (but don't lock your elbows). Lower yourself back into the pool slowly, then repeat five to 10 times.

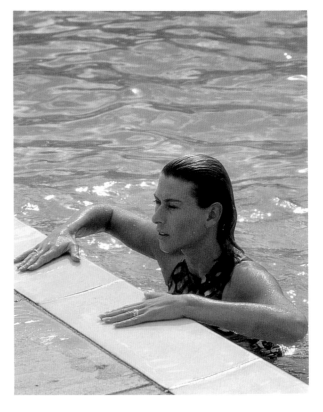

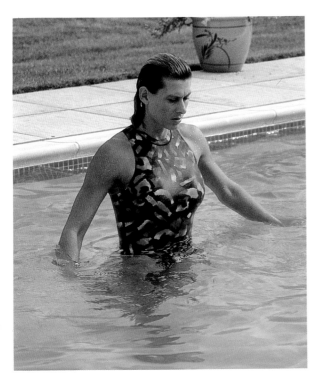
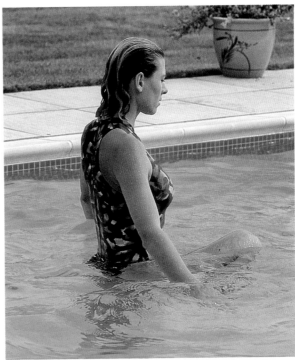
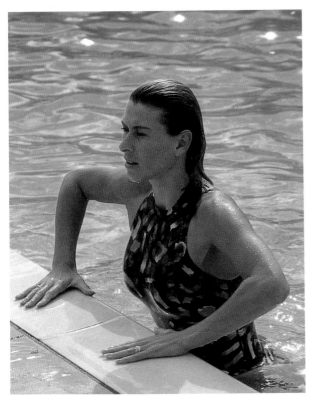
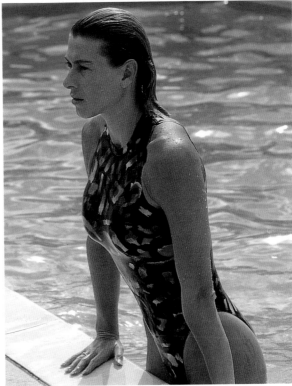

JUMPS

You need lots of space to do this energetic exercise, which is good for your legs. Be considerate of other swimmers and don't do it in a busy pool.

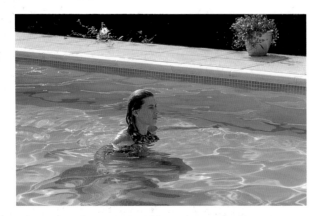

Jump up and down bringing your arms above your head and down to your sides again.

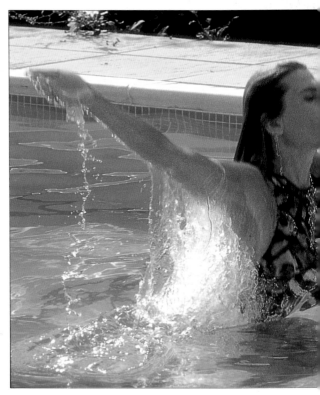

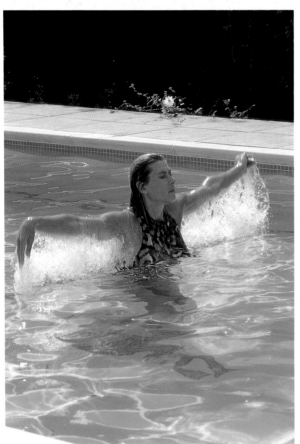

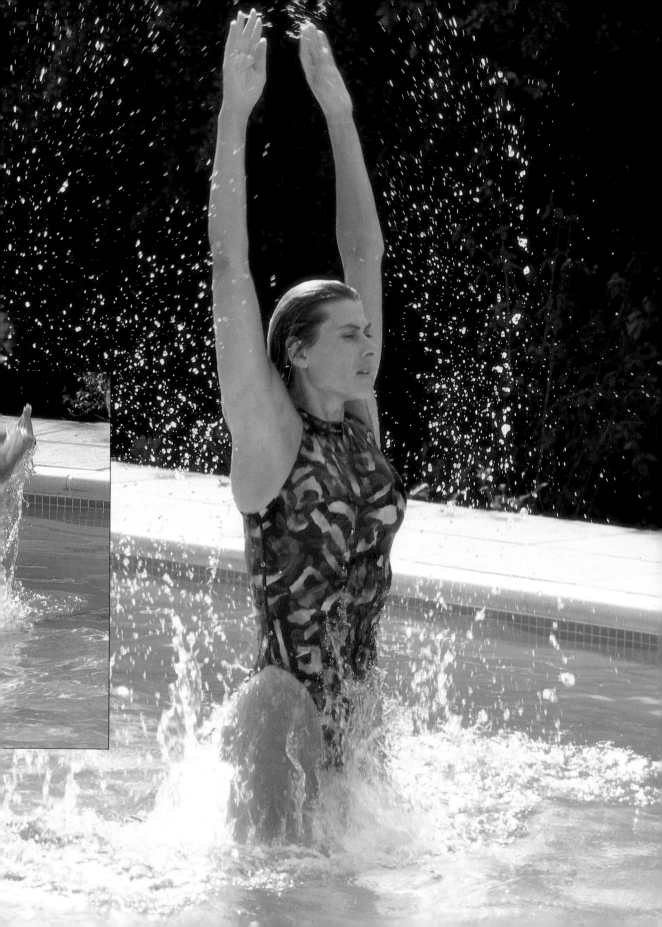

Babies and water

Young babies love the water and the sooner you introduce them to it the better. If you have your own pool you can be sure that it is clean, but with a public pool it is better to wait until your baby has had his first batch of inoculations. It is not that public pools aren't clean but they do use a lot of chemicals which might upset your baby. The first time you take your baby swimming, try to pick a time when it is fairly quiet so that he won't be frightened. Check with your pool to see when they recommend. They might even run special sessions for mums and tots, or have a separate baby pool which is warmer than the general pool. Take things very slowly at first. Don't stay in the water for more than about 15 minutes on your first visit because a tiny baby can't tell you when he is getting cold, and he can't shiver.

Of course, one way to introduce a baby to the fun that can be had in water is by playing in the bath. Make bath time a time for play and gradually get him used to getting his face wet, being lightly splashed and generally increase his confidence in the water.

Bath time can be fun, but never leave a young child alone in the bath, not even for a few seconds.

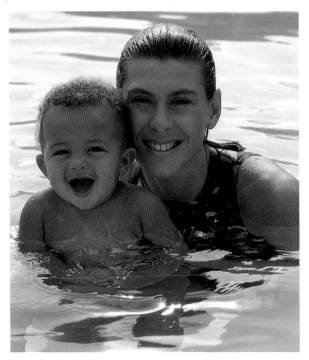

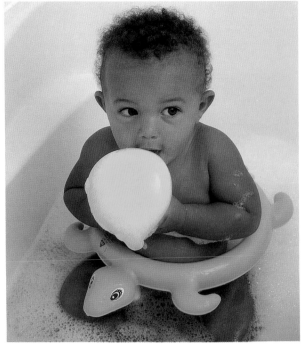

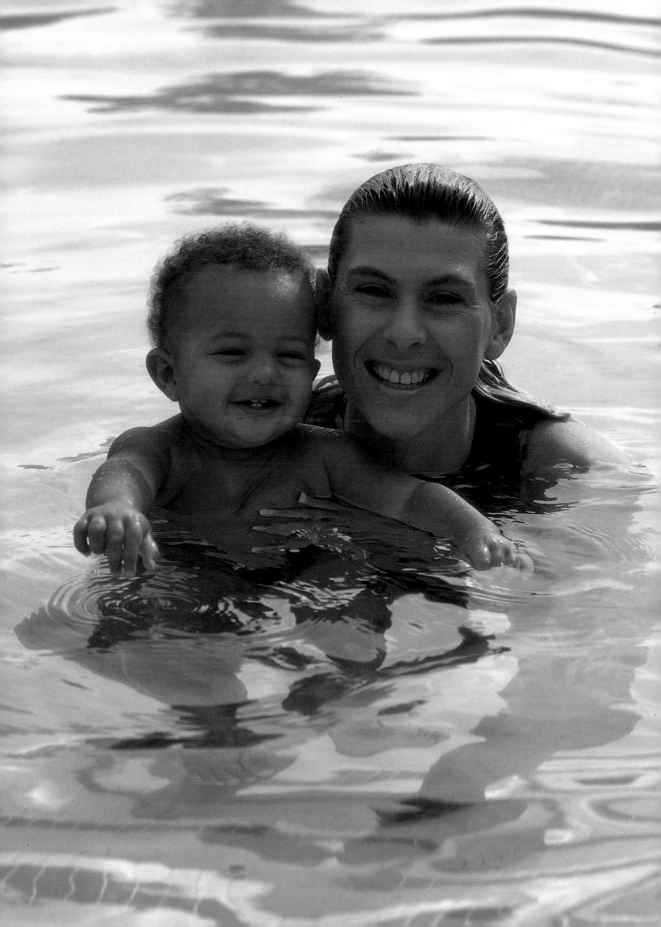

A word about Caesareans

If you had your baby delivered by Caesarian section you will be in much more pain and discomfort than if you'd had a normal delivery. Naturally this means that your approach to exercise needs to be tempered with a greater degree of caution. The best advice I can give is to be governed by what your doctor advises and to take things very gradually. Your stomach muscles will have been cut for your section, so take it *very* gently until they have repaired.

Practical matters

The first few days of a baby's life at home are likely to be rather chaotic. You will receive a visit from a midwife for the first 10 days of your baby's life, which includes those days you spend in hospital, and then care will be handed over to a health visitor who will call on you fairly regularly when you first get home, as often as you and she feel is necessary. You will have visitors dropping in to say congratulations and to bring gifts, your partner may be off from work or you may have someone else staying with you to help out. Eventually, however, you will have to settle down and fall into some sort of routine. There are all sorts of changes to cope with, from practical ones such as where to put everything, to psychological ones like bearing responsibility for a new life.

It is important that you find time to take some exercise each day, even if it is just 10 minutes – and it is surprising how difficult it can be to find 10 minutes at first. Don't forget to eat, and this is even more important if you are breastfeeding. The advice is much the same as when you were pregnant. Eat a healthy variety of food at regular intervals, and don't worry too much about dieting. If you steer clear of sugary and fatty foods and eat sensibly, then you will soon regain your normal weight. Remember that much of the surplus was baby any-way, so you won't have as far to go as you might have thought. While you are breastfeeding you should not go on a slimming diet, because you need the extra calories. You might feel flabby but some toning exercises will put this right.

It is perhaps worth mentioning here that breastfeeding will help you to return to your normal shape because as you feed your uterus contracts. This can be quite painful and I wondered what it was at first, but as soon as I had it explained to me I was glad of the pain in a perverse kind of way because I knew it was my body going back to normal.

Don't worry about housework too much. In the first few weeks people will be calling to see you and the baby not the house, so don't feel as though you have to keep everywhere pristine and have a tin of home-made biscuits at the ready to offer round. I was very lucky because my mum came to stay with me and she was able to take care of much of the housework, so that when visitors called I could enjoy their company without worrying about how the house looked. It was also lovely to have some female company, because although Derek was wonderful it was nice to have my mum to talk to as well.

It is amazing how much better a room looks just by picking things off the floor and going round with the vacuum cleaner. A laundry basket tucked behind the settee can hide a multitude of sins, too! It is rather a cliché to say 'They're not babies for long' but like most clichés it does contain a certain amount of truth, and each age has its own rewards – the tight grip of a tiny hand on your finger, the first smile, the first tentative 'Mama'. Of course it is important to keep your home clean and tidy, but if it is a lovely warm day and you have a choice between taking your baby for a walk or doing the ironing there's really no contest. Grab the sunshine while you can.

Don't forget to put in your claim for Child Benefit as soon as you can because it cannot be backdated for more than six months after a claim is received. Use the coupon in leaflet FB 8 Babies and Benefits or ask at your Social Security office for a claim form and an addressed postage-paid envelope.

Post-natal check

When your baby is six weeks old you will have to visit your GP for a post-natal check, just to make sure that all is well. This is the time to bring up any problems you have or to mention any nagging worries. It is worth remembering that most doctors are parents too, and will know exactly how you feel. There is no need to be afraid that your doctor will laugh at you or to feel embarrassed, because he or she will have heard it all before, will be unshockable, and will not be embarrassed, no matter how uncomfortable you feel talking about yourself.

So if you think you have piles, then say something! It is worth making a note of any problems or questions you have as you go through your day so that when you see your health visitor or GP you don't forget what is was you wanted to ask.

At your check you might have an internal examination to make sure that everything has gone back to where it should be, and to ensure that any stitches have healed properly, but this is often only done if you have a problem or if you ask. Your blood pressure will probably be taken, and depending on the practice at your surgery you may have blood and urine tests done too.

If you have not already been given advice on family planning that will probably be discussed. It is possible to get pregnant again before your periods return, even if you are breastfeeding, so this is a subject that needs your urgent attention. I tried the three-monthly proges-terone injection but I did not like it. I have now been fitted with a coil which suits me and my lifestyle very well. Don't forget that if you used a cap before your baby was born you will need a new one because your size and shape will have altered. Also it is not advisable to go back on the combined pill while you are breastfeeding because whatever goes into you also goes into your baby. You could use the 'mini-pill' but this needs to be taken at the same time every day – not as easy as it sounds when you have so many new distractions. This is a complex subject because there are so many different contraceptives available now, and new ones are constantly being developed, so take advice on what is the best for you.

Going back to work

Going back out to work can be more demanding than you might imagine. For one thing, your mind is likely to be half on your job and half wondering if your baby is all right, at least for the first few days. But if you are confident in the child-minder or nursery care that you have arranged and can assure yourself that your child is being well looked after you will soon settle back into your old role.

It is very tiring trying to do a full day's work and then coming home to cook a meal and look after the house, perhaps having stopped off at the supermarket on the way. The logistics can be quite complex, and you could be forgiven for thinking that you are on the go all day and every day. But if you want to work, or need to for financial reasons, your baby will not suffer. Even so, if you find that leaving your baby is just too upsetting for you and you really can't concentrate, then don't be afraid to admit that you were wrong and give in your notice. No one expects you to be Wonder Woman (except possibly you) so don't try to be all things to all people.

I used to be amazed by sports people who turned down the opportunity to compete in the Commonwealth Games or the Olympics because they could not bear to be away from their children. Now, though, I understand what they meant. I found that although I am happy to train away from Elliott, racing competitively was a different matter because I couldn't concentrate properly. My priorities had changed completely and I didn't enjoy being away from him for two or three days at a time.

Relationships

You can get so wrapped up in a new baby that you forget that you also have a partner to consider. With a youngster sapping all your strength – literally, if you are breastfeeding – it is hard to keep something back for the two of you but it is vital that you do. Try to set aside some 'quality time' when you can just be a couple again for a little while. Family and friends can be enormously useful here and can babysit for a hour or so to allow you to have a meal in peace, to go for a walk, see a film, or just sit and look at each other. Make the effort to go out once a month, or you will forget how to.

If you don't have anyone living nearby whom you can leave your baby with, investigate babysitting circles. These are excellent because members sit for one another in return for tokens worth one hour's time rather than hard cash. If there isn't one near you, why not set one up? Some of the organisations listed at the back of the book can help you here, or talk to your health visitor because she often knows who is involved in circles.

If all else fails, there are lots of 'grown-up' things you can do with a baby in tow. Many restaurants are happy to have children in, particularly at lunchtime, so just pack up your pushchair and go. A lot will even have highchairs, but a useful purchase I have made is a portable highchair that can clip on to the edge of any table. You can also get a

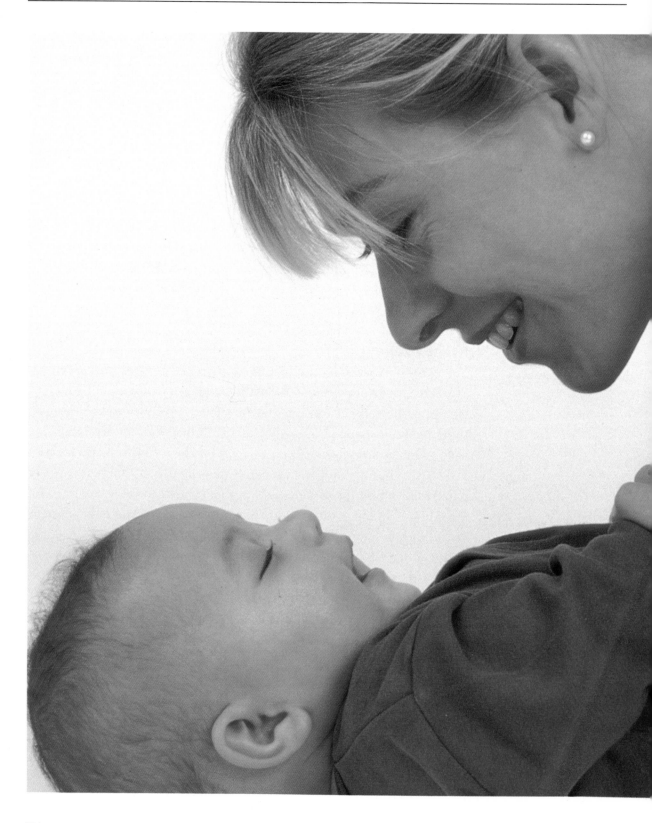

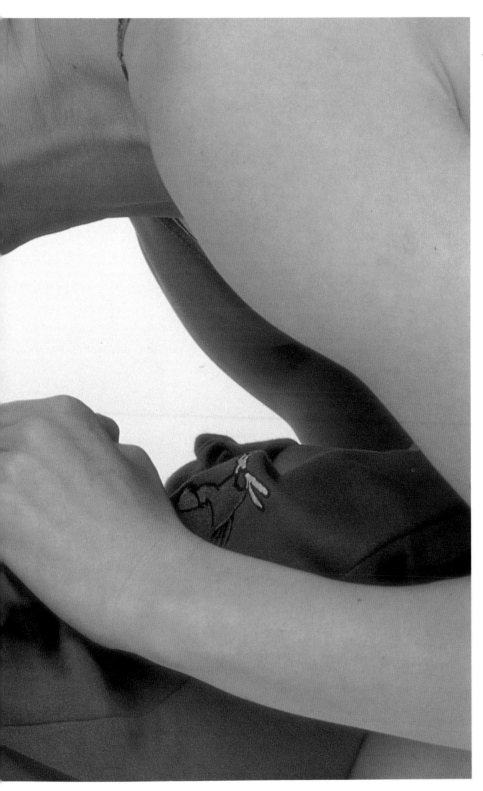

*'I was amazed at
just how much joy
Elliott brought into
our lives.'*

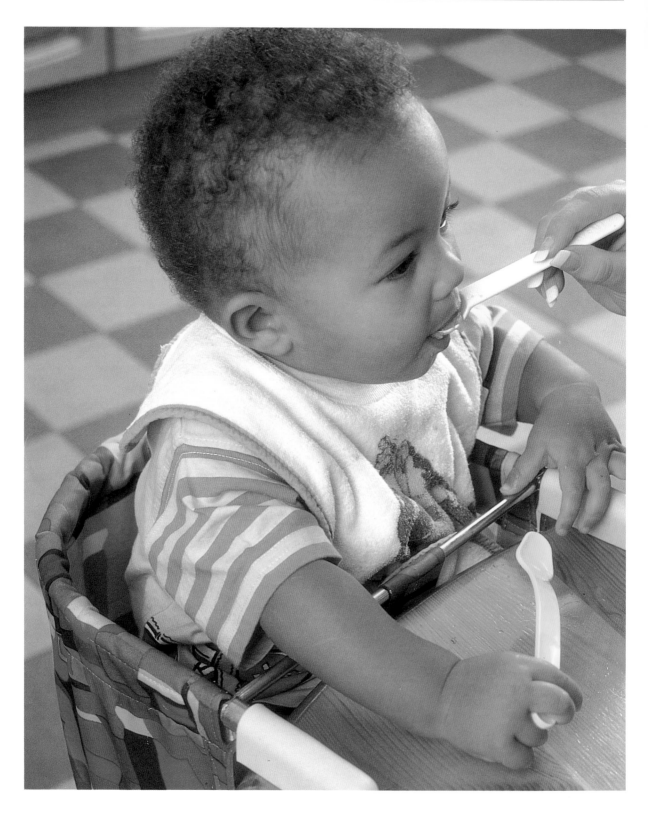

Many restaurants provide high chairs, but if they don't a portable high chair can prove to be a useful investment for when you are out and about.

light version which fastens around a chair. When the baby is very young the chances are he will just sleep all the time you are out anyway, or if not it often only takes a feed to settle him. If you fancy a drink, choose a pub with a family room which is likely to be less smoky than a public bar, or better still sit in the beer garden. What about a lunchtime concert, where etiquette is likely to be more relaxed than for an evening performance? Go to a gallery or museum; visit a country park you have never been to before; go window shopping; visit a stately home; browse round a garden centre and have a cream tea in the café; check if your local authority organises guided walks around your area: these are often free or at least inexpensive and many are suitable for pushchairs. If not you could carry the child in a backpack. You will find that the more you take a baby out – and this is equally true of older children – the more you *can* take him out. There are lots of things you can do, so there is no reason to feel trapped in the house or to give up your social life altogether. It is just a matter of adapting to your new circumstances, and planning ahead rather more than you had to when there was just the two of you and you could go off somewhere at a moment's notice.

Make time for yourself

With all the effort you are making to tend to the needs of the family, don't forget that you are special, too. Don't feel guilty if you put your feet up and watch a soap opera for half an hour while the baby is asleep. It is easy to say and not so easy to do, but try to make time to do something that is just for you. Sit in the garden and browse through a magazine, have your hair cut, visit a friend: really anything that makes you feel good is worth while – and if you need to justify it to yourself, remember that if you are not well and happy then neither will your family be.

Older children

Even the most well-adjusted youngster is likely to be a little unsettled by the arrival of a new baby, so you must do all you can to ensure that the transition from only child to big brother or sister is as smooth as possible. Not every child is bound to be jealous of a new arrival, but if it happens it is very upsetting for everyone. Nevertheless it needs to be

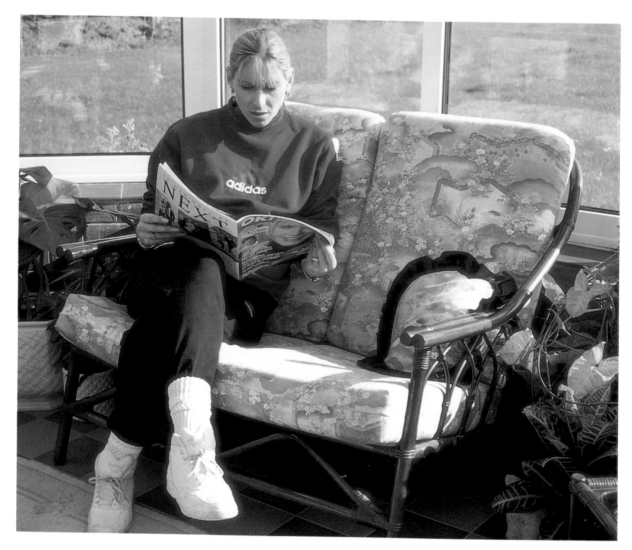

dealt with. It is another of those aspects of parenting that everyone has an opinion on, how to avoid it, what to do if it occurs.

If you think your older child is showing signs of resentment get advice from your health visitor. He may start reverting to babyish habits like crying for attention, wanting a bottle instead of a beaker, wetting the bed, being clingy, not wanting to be left with other people, or the jealousy may come out in uncharacteristic behaviour, such as suddenly becoming unusually boisterous, stubborn, or violent, perhaps even lashing out at the new baby.

Try to make time to spend just with your older child doing the things you used to do before the baby was born, but don't exclude

It can be hard to find time just to sit and read a magazine for a while but do try to because you deserve the rest.

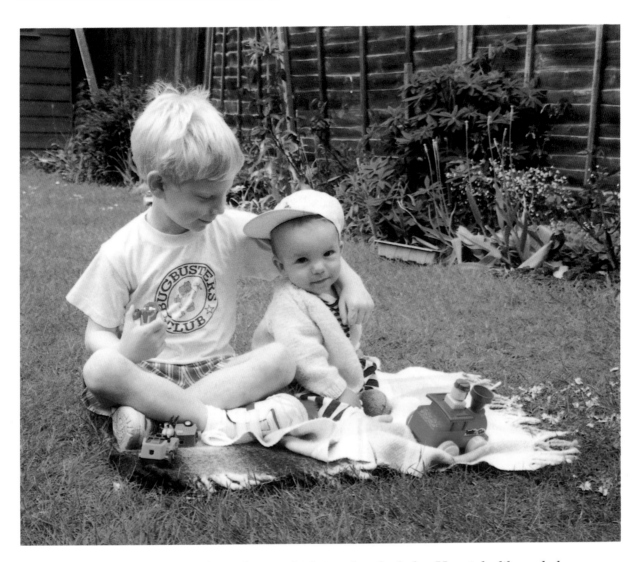

The Thorley boys, Sam and Joe, are the best of friends.

Photograph: Julia Thorley.

him from things which involve the baby. He might like to help you bath him or fetch clothes for you, but if he doesn't want to don't make a fuss. Don't push him either towards the baby or away, but try to look for the signs and help him adjust in the way he wants to. At the same time try to maintain the old routine as far as possible, so that your child has something familiar to reassure him that everything is all right.

One tip that was passed on to Julia was for the new baby to 'buy' a present for his big brother or sister. So the first time Sam went to see baby Joe in hospital there was present waiting for him, and he is very proud of the watch that 'my baby brother gave me'.

Chapter 9

YOUR PARTNER

This chapter is written for you, but you might also want to give it to your partner to read. Books and magazines for women are everywhere, but it is not so easy for men to get the information they need. They might feel that the questions they want to ask are stupid, or that it is not very macho to show more than a passing interest in your pregnancy. They might just feel scared and confused. But just as you want him to support you, you must try to help him. After all, it is his baby too and he will probably be there for the birth, so he needs to know what is going on.

There is as big an assumption today that your partner will want to be at the birth as there was 20 years ago that he *wouldn't* want to be there. The thought of seeing the woman he loves in great pain, and being subjected to all manner of medical care – not to mention all that blood and gore! – is enough to make even the strongest man have a few qualms. In fact, fathers in attendance rarely do actually faint or throw up. Generally they are so swept along by the excitement and emotion of the occasion that they don't even notice the messy bits. Derek had said that he was not going to look at what was happening at the 'business end', but was going to content himself with holding my hand and murmuring words of encouragement. In the event he was keen to see the baby's head when it first appeared, and after the birth he was on hand with the camera so that every moment was recorded for posterity. Even so, if your partner is feeling nervous about being present, don't make a big thing about it. Just like you, he needs to gather all the information about him and make up his own mind. It can often help to talk to other dads who have been through it for reassurance that it really isn't all that bad.

Before the birth
There is a lot that your partner can do to help you before the birth of

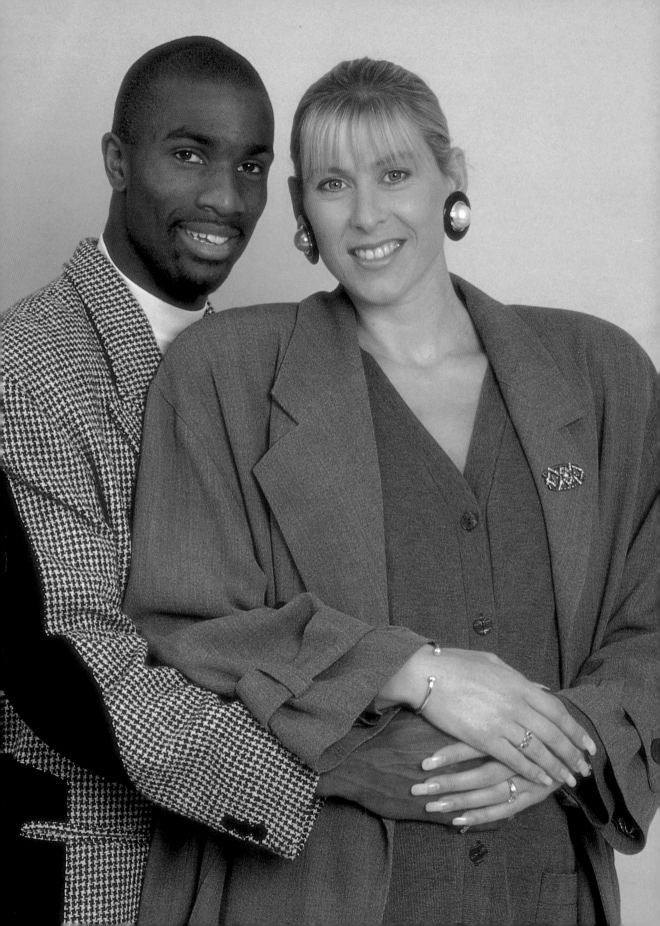

your baby – as long as you tell him what it is you want. You can't expect him to be psychic. I appreciate that it might be difficult for him to arrange time off work to attend at antenatal classes or routine appointments with you, but if he can so much the better. If he can manage to go with you when you have a scan, that is lovely because seeing the baby on the monitor will move even the most stern of male hearts. I was very glad that Derek could be with me. At some ante-natal classes dads are encouraged to join in the exercises and to practise the breathing, which is very useful later on when you come to your labour.

At the end of this chapter I have given some suggestions of ante-natal exercises that your partner can do with you.

Your man also has a very valuable job to do in boosting your ego. Every mum-to-be needs to be regularly reassured that she is still a person in her own right, not just a baby carrier. You need someone to tell you that you look gorgeous, that you are still sexy. You will also need him to be more than usually understanding as your mood swings from one extreme to the other, so during your saner moments explain to him why you are sometimes rather *insane*. You could warn him, too, that you are likely to be transformed during your labour from the mild, sweet-natured women he knows and loves to a screaming alien, and that if you tell him you hate him and never want to see him again you don't really mean it. I never felt like this but I do know of women who did.

There is no need to put an end to your sex life just because you are expecting a baby. In fact a lot of women say they feel particularly amorous while they are pregnant. Assure your partner that your baby is well protected inside you and he cannot harm it, and then enjoy experimenting with different positions that are satisfying and com-fortable for you both. The 'spoons' position is a favourite with many expectant couples.

I borrowed lots of videos about childbirth while I was pregnant because I wanted to be aware of everything that could happen. Derek didn't want to see them because he said the only baby he wanted to see born was his own, but some dads might be interested to see them so that there are no surprises.

On a more practical level you could write some lists of things that

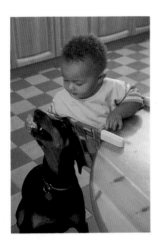

Elliott and the family dog Bella.

will need doing while you are in hospital, such as who to ring, what to do with your other children if you have any, how to keep the house going in your absence. You should also delegate to him the job of cleaning up after your dog and emptying the cat litter tray because of the risk of toxoplasmosis. A parasite lives in the intestine of these animals which can cause an infection in humans. An adult might develop flu-like symptoms, but any infection in pregnancy might lead to miscarriage, stillbirth or brain damage. In children it can cause blindness.

During labour

It is a good idea for your partner to familiarise himself with the jargon of pregnancy and birth, so that in the heat of the moment he will understand what is being said and can let you know what is happening if you are not sure what is going on, and tell you who the strange faces are if someone new comes into the room. He needs to be familiar with your birth plan, and to be prepared to make decisions on your behalf if you are not able to speak for yourself for some reason. I always consulted with Derek about my antenatal care and my wishes for labour, and he just agreed with whatever I wanted. However, if he had violently objected to something I would have listened to his point of view and done what I could to accommodate his wishes.

I have heard several dads say that they felt useless during the birth of their child because while mum was lying there doing all the work they had nothing to do except watch. It can be frightening to see the one you love in pain and not be able to do anything to stop it. You must reassure your man that he mustn't underestimate the importance of simply being there, sharing the moment. I wouldn't have wanted to go through it without Derek at my side and just knowing that he was with me gave me great encouragement, and made me feel safe. I didn't let him sleep while I was having contractions so at the end of it all he was tired too, and better placed to understand how I felt.

In fact there are some practical things he can do for you during your labour. If you are using a TENS machine, he can put it on for you. He can massage your back, let you lean on him, hold on very tight during the strongest part of the contractions let you dig your

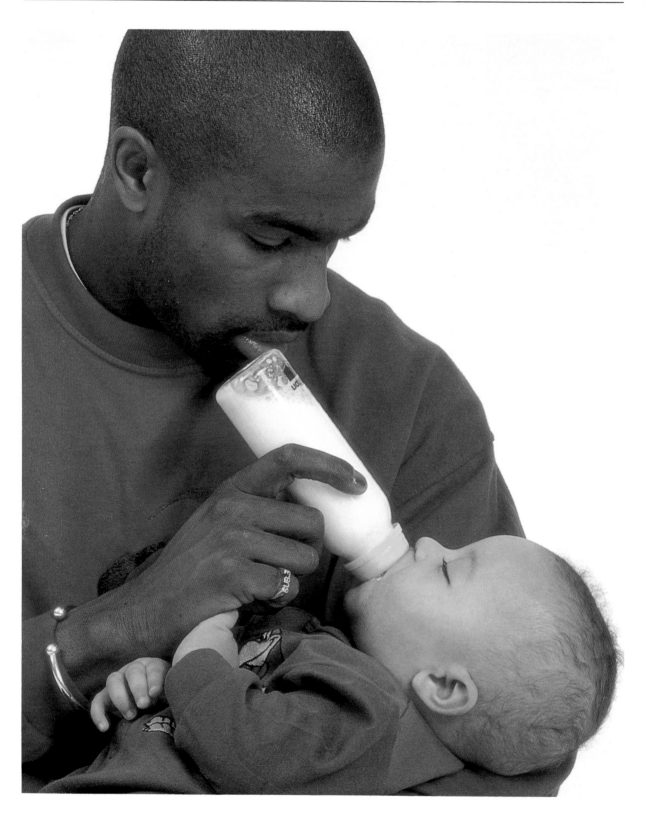

nails into him, if needs be, wipe your face, get you a drink, talk to you and sooth you, remind you to breathe properly – yes, I know you think this is a silly thing to say, but believe me you need reminding!

Elliott was given to Derek almost as soon as he was born and he held him while I was stitched, and Julia's husband Clive was given both their children straight away, too.

After the birth

Your partner will be almost as worried as you about how you will react to being a mother. The transition from couple to family is quite dramatic and takes some getting used to. The best thing you can do is to put aside your preconceptions and let things develop naturally.

Today looking after a child is generally accepted to be part of the role of both parents, not just mum. Dads are quite capable of changing nappies, preparing food, playing (especially playing). I feel that since Derek and I both made Elliott we have joint responsibility for

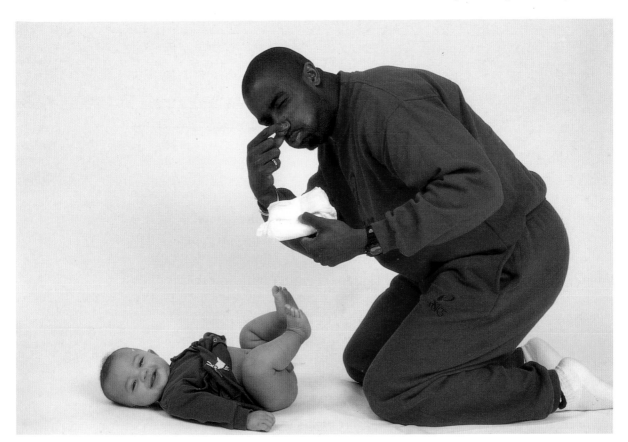

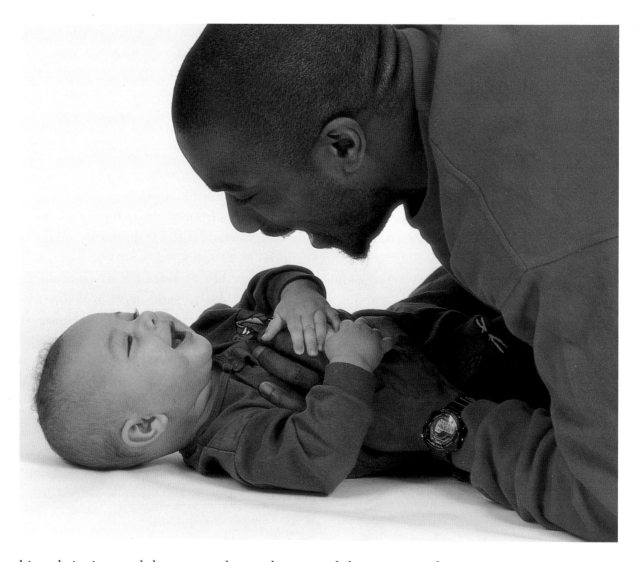

his upbringing, and that means the good parts and the not so good. Derek knows Elliott as well as I do, and because I know he can cope without me I am confident in his ability to look after him. The only thing he doesn't do is to buy Elliott's clothes; he hasn't quite got the eye for the sizes.

Reassure your man that it is all right to show his feelings, to be 'soft' when it comes to his children. Encourage him to talk about his worries and hopes. A problem that is aired is halfway to being solved. If you suffer from the baby blues and are tearful, you will need your partner to support you. It will help him though if he realises that this is a normal post-natal reaction and that most women experience it as their hormones are still in a state of flux. It is not helped if you are always tired and anxious, so try to rest whenever you can and let Dad take over for a while. If these feelings go on and on for weeks, however, and you feel really down, you might be suffering from more serious post-natal depression and will need medical help, so talk to your doctor.

Some men experience a bit of jealousy towards their new baby because of the amount of time their partner spends with him and the close bond that is formed. They might also find it uncomfortable to see you breastfeeding at first. Be aware that this might happen and make sure that you do not exclude your man. Save some intimate moments for him, too. He (and you) might be hesitant about resuming a sex life, but take things gently and you will soon be back to normal. You might be a little sore and tentative at first, particularly if you have had stitches or an especially traumatic delivery, so ask your partner to be patient. If you find sex very painful, talk to your doctor.

Exercises you can do together

STRETCH I

This stretch is good fun, but must be done gently so as not to strain your back. It will work on your hamstrings and your bottom.

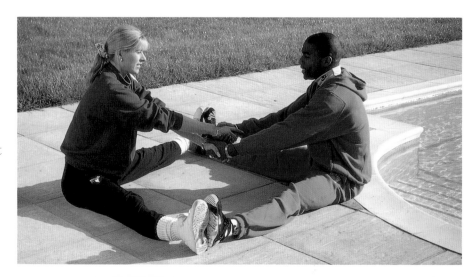

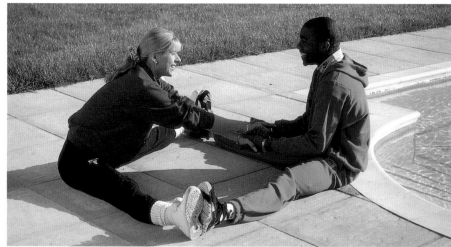

Sit with your legs as far apart as is comfortable for you. Your partner should sit in a similar position facing you with his feet either touching or tucked inside yours. Keep your knees on the floor, look forwards and keep your back straight. Let your partner gently pull you towards him as far as is comfortable. Repeat this three to five times.

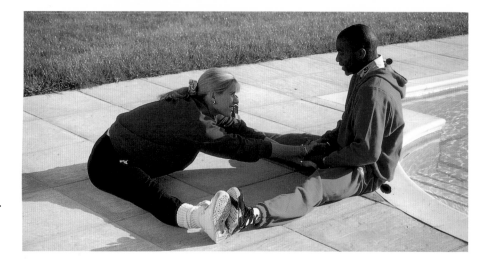

STRETCH 2

If you are doing this stretch correctly you should feel it working on your inner thighs, but it should not become painful.

Sit with the soles of your feet together and your back straight. Your partner should crouch behind you and gently push your knees towards the floor. Repeat three to five times.

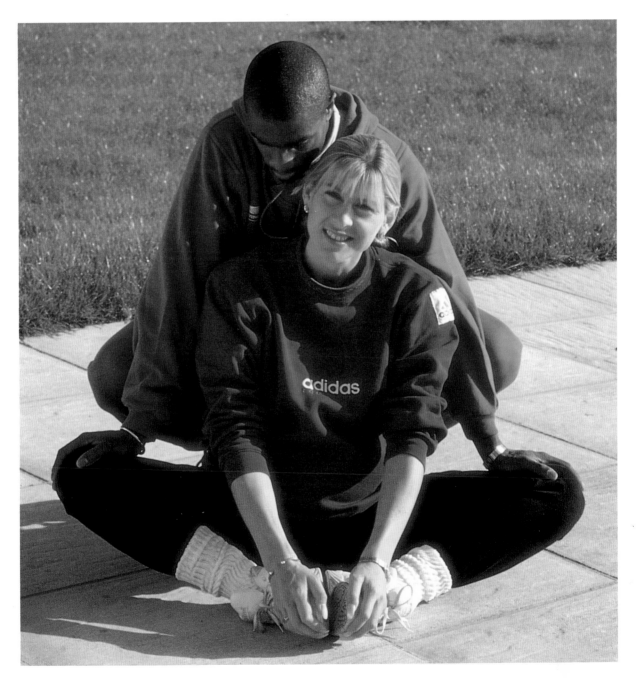

STRETCH 3

This simple exercise will really work your bottom and thighs.

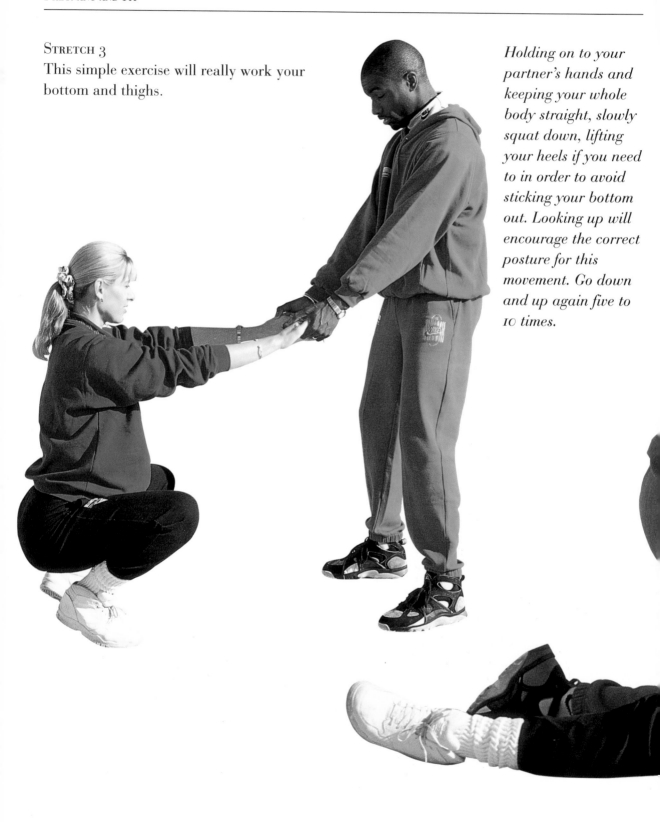

Holding on to your partner's hands and keeping your whole body straight, slowly squat down, lifting your heels if you need to in order to avoid sticking your bottom out. Looking up will encourage the correct posture for this movement. Go down and up again five to 10 times.

STRETCH 4

This is not as difficult as it looks because your partner supports the weight of your leg. Don't worry if you can't raise your leg to a right angle. Just go as far as is comfortable. You should feel a stretch all the way down the back of your raised leg, ie your bottom, your hamstring and your calf muscles.

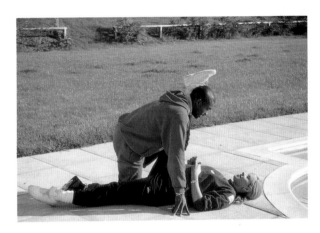

Lie with your legs apart so that your partner can kneel on one knee with that knee between your legs and the foot of his other leg flat on the floor outside your legs, so that he can support your raised leg on his shoulder. While he holds your knee, flex your foot. Repeat 3-5 times on each leg.

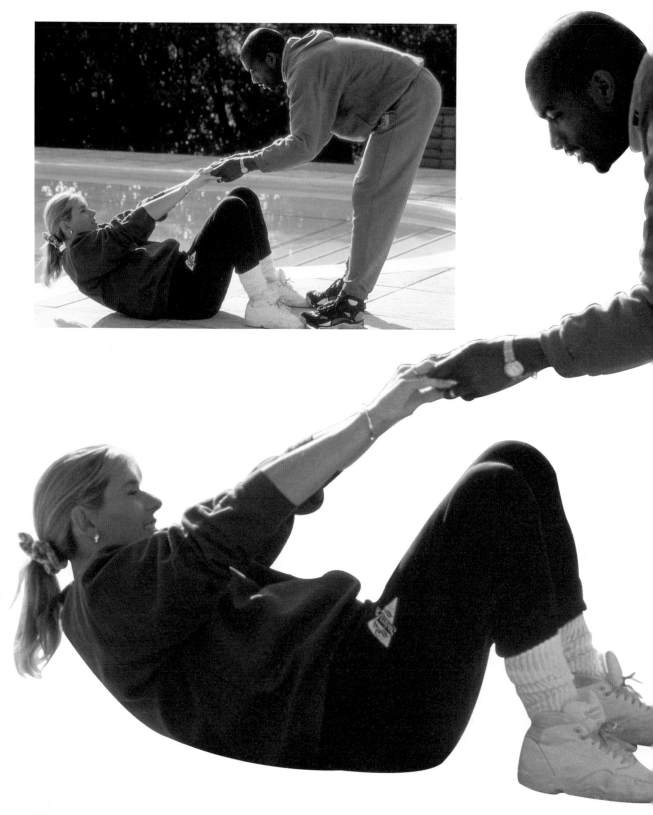

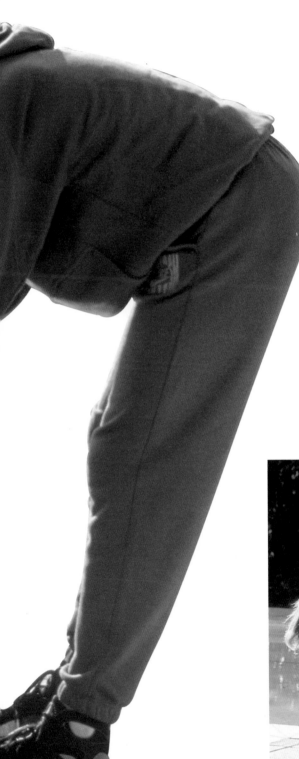

SUPPORTED SIT-UP

This is a variation on the conventional sit-up and it is safe to do because your partner supports some of your weight. The amount of help he gives you will depend on your strength. Don't strain, just go as far you feel comfortable. This exercise works on the front of your thighs and your tummy muscles.

Lie with your knees bent and your back flat on the floor. Your partner should stand on your toes (gently!) and pull you towards him so that you go through the movements of a sit-up but with him doing some of the work. Repeat 10 to 20 times to suit.

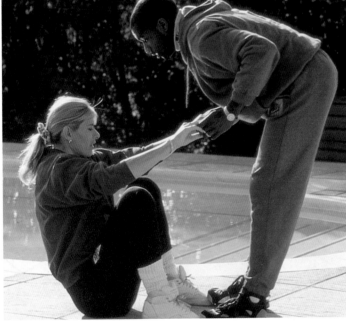

LEG RAISE

The start of this exercise is the hard part. Once you have raised your leg past the 45° point the rest is easy! As well as the front of your thighs, this will also work your stomach muscles, including those down the side (the obliques).

Lie on your back with your partner behind you, and hold on to his legs so that you are firmly anchored. Bend one knee, then slowly raise the opposite leg as far as you can, then lower it to the floor again with equal control. Repeat three to five times on each side.

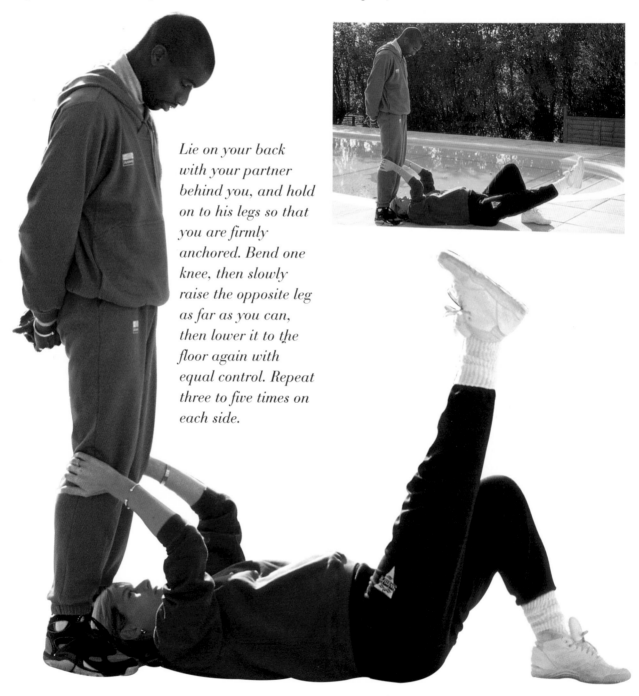

Exercises that work your stomach muscles, like the last two, should be executed carefully and dropped altogether towards the end of your pregnancy. If you have back problems or weak stomach muscles you can do the leg raise, but bend your knees and only lift your leg halfway. These exercises are especially good for getting your stomach back into shape after your baby is born.

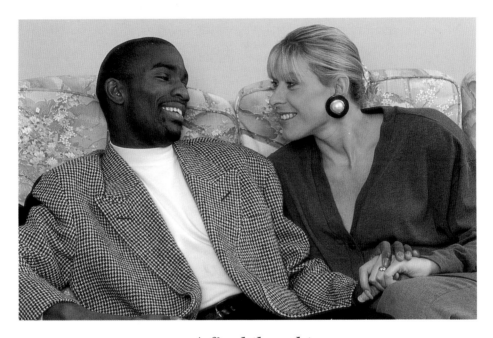

A final thought

Amid all the excitement of having a new baby, don't forget to say 'I love you' to each other just once in a while.

USEFUL INFORMATION

List of useful addresses

Many of these organisations are registered charities, so if writing please enclosed an sae.

Active Birth Centre
55 Dartmouth Park Road
London NW5 1SL
0171 267 3006

Association of Breastfeeding
Mothers
10 Herschell Road
London SE23 1EG
0181 778 4769

Association for Improvements in
the Maternity Services
21 Iver Lane
Iver
Bucks SL0 9LH
01753 652781

Association for Post-natal Illness
25 Jerdan Place
London SW6 1BE
0171 386 0868

Association of Radical Midwives
62 Greetby Hill
Ormskirk
Lancs L39 2DT
01695 572776

British Diabetic Association
10 Queen Anne Street
London
W1M 0BD
0171 323 1531

British Pregnancy Advisory
Service
Austy Manor
Wotton Wawen
Solihull
West Midlands B95 6BS
01564 793225

Caesarian Support Network
c/o Mrs Tunstall
2 Hurst Park Drive
Huyton
Merseyside L36 1TF
0151 480 1184

Down's Syndrome Association
155 Mitcham Road
London SW17 9PG
0181 682 4001

Independent Midwives Association
94 Auckland Road
London SE19 2DB

La Lèche League of Great Britain
BM3424
London WC1N 3XX
0171 242 1278

Maternity Alliance
15 Britannia Street
London WC1X 9JP
(No phone calls, please)

Meet-a-Mum Association
Cornerstone House
14 Willis Road
Croydon
SR0 2XX
0181 665 0357

Miscarriage Association
c/o Clayton Hospital
Northgate
Wakefield
West Yorkshire WF1 3JS
01924 200799

National Childbirth Trust
Alexandra House
Oldham Terrace
London W3 6NH
0181 992 8637

National Council for One Parent
Families
255 Kentish Town Road
London NW5 2LX
0171 267 1361

Royal College of Midwives
15 Mansfield Street
London W1
0171 580 6523

Things you will need to take into hospital with you

Your hospital will probably give you a list of essential items that you will need during your stay, and this is likely to vary considerably depending on where you have your confinement. Some hospitals need you to provide everything from sanitary towels to clothes for your baby. Some wards encourage you to get dressed during your stay, while others prefer you to stay in your dressing-gown and slippers. You won't have a lot of room to store things, so don't overdo it and be guided by the list provided by the hospital.

FOR YOUR LABOUR

Any paperwork your hospital may have requested you bring, including your notes.

- Sanitary towels – if your waters break early you will need these. Take in at least two dozen either special maternity pads or maxi-absorbency ordinary pads. Don't underestimate the number or absorbency you will need.
- Food for your partner – the NHS does not run to providing nourishment for non-participants! You might also want to take some squash for yourself and perhaps some high-energy foods to keep yourself going, such as dried fruit or glucose tablets. I was told not to eat in case I needed a general anaesthetic, but instead was advised to take a vacuum flask full of ice-cubes with me, which I found soothing to suck.
- TENS machine – if appropriate, plus any other equipment you plan to use for pain relief.
- Flannel – to mop your fevered brow.
- Atomiser – to refresh yourself.
- Something to read – there can be a lot of hanging around so go prepared.
- Camera and video recorder (if allowed).

DURING YOUR STAY

- Three nightdresses, front-fastening if you are breastfeeding.
- Nursing bras and breast pads.
- Nipple cream.
- Sanitary pads (and make sure you have an extra supply in at home).

- Disposable nappies. Even if you intend to use terry nappies when you get home you will have to use disposable ones in hospital. It is now possible to buy special nappies for newborn babies that have a shaped front that helps to keep the cord dry.
- Light dressing gown and cardigan to wear as a bed jacket.
- A small amount of change to buy a newspaper, make phone calls etc (and don't forget your address book).
- Cotton wool.
- Tissues.
- Your toiletries and make-up.
- Two large bath towels.
- Soft toilet tissue.
- Disposable pants.

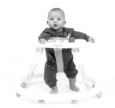

Baby walker.

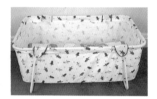

Travel cot.

COMING HOME

(these things can be brought in for you by your partner on the day you leave)

- Something for you to wear. You will be smaller than you were when you went in but not yet ready for your pre-bump clothes. Those trusty leggings are useful yet again . . .
- Something for your baby to wear. As well as a nappy, he should wear three layers – vest, suit and cardigan – plus a shawl which covers his head as well as his body.
- Car seat. It is illegal to carry a baby in a car without it being restrained, so make sure you are prepared either by having properly anchored straps for a carry-cot or by fitting a seat. Many hospitals operate a hire service.

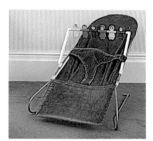

Carrying sling.

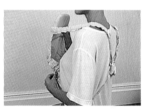

Bouncy chair.

Nursery equipment

Not all of the following items are essential, and what you buy will depend largely on your lifestyle, your budget and how much room you have to store things. The following list covers just about everything you might need, but much of it is optional. For instance you don't have to buy a baby bath. You can put your baby in the full-size bath straight away as long as you are confident and careful, or put him in the bath with you or your partner. One advantage of a baby bath is that it can be put on a stand or firm table so that you do not have to bend so far.

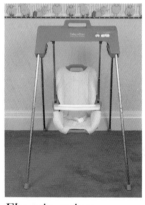

Electric swing.

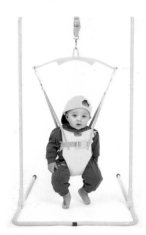

Elliott has been 'upright' from an early age, both in a bouncing frame here and in his baby walker. I think that this may have contributed to his being able to walk at eight months.

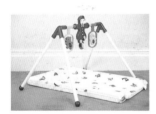

Changing mat with play gym.

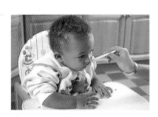

High chair.

- Moses bed or baby nest.
- Cot.
- Three sets of cot sheets.
- Two cot blankets.
- Carrycot.
- Travel cot.
- Pram or pushchair with waterproof covers and sunshade.
- Stroller.
- Carrying sling.
- Cat/insect net.
- Playpen.
- Two dozen terry nappies with liners, safety lock nappy pins and plastic pants, or disposable nappies.
- Nappy sacks.

- Nappy bin.
- Baby wipes.
- Changing mat.
- Changing bag.
- Cotton wool.
- Baby lotion.
- Baby bath.
- Baby bubble bath or soap.
- Baby shampoo.
- Baby cream.
- Baby powder (although some people advise against this because babies can breathe it in).
- Round-ended scissors (or clippers which are easier to use).
- Box for all the bits and pieces.

- Bottles and sterilising equipment.
- Breast pump.
- Chest of drawers.
- Activity centre.
- Mobile.
- Baby listening device.
- Car seat.
- Bouncy chair.
- Electric swing.
- Baby walker.
- Bouncer.
- Safety equipment, eg cupboard locks, fridge lock, stair gate, fire guard, covers for sharp corners, film to cover glass doors, socket covers.

Clothes for your baby

Don't buy a lot of first size clothes, because they only fit for a very short time and are the size that people will give you as gifts. To get you started you will need the following:

- Four vests.
- Half a dozen suits which can be worn day or night.
- Three cardigans (not necessarily woolly matinee coats if you feel these are rather old-fashioned; choose something in sweatshirt-style fabric).
- Outdoor coat or large shawl or padded all-in-one.
- Hat.
- Socks or bootees.

INDEX